Growing Healthy Children

A Framework for Understanding Health

ELLEN D. ALLEN, ND

THIS BOOK SHOULD NOT BE USED TO DIAGNOSE OR TREAT MEDICAL CONDITIONS OR DISEASES.

Growing Healthy Children © 2005 by Ellen D. Allen. All rights reserved. No part of this book may be reproduced in any manner whatsoever without written permission, except in the case of brief quotations embedded in critical articles and reviews.

Published by:
RubyFire
P.O. Box 727
Highlands, TX 77562-0727
www.rubyfire.net

Cover design by Artlink
Book design by Sara Patton

Printed in the United States of America
ISBN 13: 978-0-978642-10-5
ISBN 10: 0-978642-10-4

Contents

CHAPTER 1	Understanding Health	1
CHAPTER 2	Happy, Healthy Children	5
CHAPTER 3	Individual Differences	11
CHAPTER 4	Growth and Development: My World	17
CHAPTER 5	Structure and Function	31
CHAPTER 6	Too Much, Too Little	41
CHAPTER 7	Assessment	53
CHAPTER 8	Systems Overview	59
CHAPTER 9	Nutrition	67
CHAPTER 10	Protection: The Immune System	79
CHAPTER 11	Communication: The Neuroendocrine System	89
CHAPTER 12	Detoxification	95
CHAPTER 13	Stress: The Driving Force in Life	103
CHAPTER 14	Wiser Choices	113
EPILOGUE	A Job Well Done	117
GLOSSARY		119
REFERENCES AND AUTHOR'S NOTES		123

Editor's Note

Mary Conrad Lo, MD
Wilmington, DE, USA
July 2005

It has been my pleasure to edit the first of a series of books by Ellen Allen, ND, which will present, among many other things, some novel techniques that she has developed in her clinic for children in Australia. These techniques utilize the concept of "bioresonance," or energy, and will be discussed elsewhere in the series.

This book is full of wisdom—full of grace. Through stories and simple but striking illustrations, it introduces Ellen's integrated view of life, which encompasses a more complete definition of health than is often encountered in our modern clinical world. Recommendations for achieving optimal function are introduced along with some basic instruction in how the human body works.

The material in this book has not been subjected to the level of editorial scrutiny normally provided for peer-reviewed journal entries or medical textbooks. *This book should not be used to diagnose or treat medical conditions.* Many references have been provided to facilitate further research by the reader.

The fields of nutrition as therapy and environmental medicine are in early stages of development; therefore much in both of these areas remains to be proven in the normal, scientific sense, and may be considered experimental, or even speculative, by many in conventional medicine. Some of these individuals also tend to question the merits of acupuncture and homeopathy—the two established energy therapies in use for many years throughout the world—and other "complementary" therapies. In turn, speculation regarding the value of much of conventional medicine exists on the part of many "alternative" therapists. Increasingly there are signs of cooperation and a willingness to explore other points of view. Such efforts can only benefit those who suffer illness.

Unsettling as it may be, our collective knowledge, and what we believe to be true, is continually changing. A recent study has shown that when "all original clinical research studies published in three major general clinical journals or high-impact-factor specialty journals in 1990–2003 and cited more than 1,000 times in the literature were examined . . . 7 (16%) were contradicted by subsequent studies, 7 others (16%) had found effects that were stronger than those of subsequent studies, 20 (44%) were replicated, and 11 (24%) remained largely unchallenged." [John P. A. Ioannidis, MD, "Contradicted and Initially Stronger Effects in Highly Cited Clinical Research," *JAMA* 2005; 294:218–228.]

My experiences—in basic science research, clinical allopathic medicine, classical homeopathy, and, in no small measure, the editing of this book—have led me to formulate a view of our collective knowledge regarding the nature of life, and the processes we use to develop our beliefs. I can include in this view a few kinds of health care systems with which I have some familiarity. I can best represent this view as a continuous circular spectrum using color, forming an analogy to the color wheel (as opposed to the linear spectrum of light). (Note: "Allopathic" means "different from" and refers to the usual type of pharmaceutical medicine.)

ORANGE
- Physics (mathematics)
- Biochemistry

RED
- Genomics
- Human biology and physiology
- Medical research—allopathic
- Firmly established allopathic medical practice

EDITOR'S NOTE

PURPLE
- Developing fields in allopathic medicine
  - Environmental medicine
  - Nutrition as therapy

BLUE
- "Alternative" traditions in which natural substances are used in an allopathic way
  - Naturopathy (includes some use of homeopathic remedies in an allopathic way)
  - Native American medicine
  - Traditional Chinese medicine

GREEN
- Emerging energy or "bioresonance" therapies
  - Ellen's developing techniques
- Firmly established energy therapies
  - Acupuncture
  - Classical homeopathy
- Meditation/prayer/kundalini yoga (somehow connected to health and energy)

YELLOW
- Energy itself: Whatever it is that leaves the body, or ceases to operate, when we die: the Essence of Life: the Spirit.

Although all do both, subatomic, atomic, and molecular science (orange), and the therapies shown under green predominantly influence or concern the domain of energy; the life sciences and allopathic therapies (red, purple, and blue) predominantly influence or concern the realm of matter. When visualized on a color wheel, each line would have its own color since each is different, making a smooth, continuous transition around a full circle.

Keep in mind that at a subatomic level, the distinction between matter and energy becomes quite blurred.

In my view, energy therapists attempt to manipulate what some experimental physicists may one day at least partially elucidate. Both approach the essence of life itself—from opposite directions. In my opinion, the exact nature of energy is something that will remain a mystery.

I have no knowledge of, or experience with, details of the energy techniques that Ellen has developed. I therefore look forward to satisfying my curiosity about these as her next books continue to reveal a body of knowledge accumulated over many years of research and experience. I certainly also expect to continue to benefit from frequent gifts to the reader of gems of insight, which provide glimpses into a solid, workable philosophy based on love, respect, and a deep sense of awe regarding the wonder that is Life.

Mary Conrad Lo, MD is a licensed physician (Maryland, USA) who has worked in basic research in two prominent medical schools and a branch of the NIH in the USA. She has undertaken formal training in classical homeopathy, and works as a freelance editor, writer, and French-to-English translator in the state of Delaware, USA, where she resides.

1

Understanding Health

Health is so much more than the absence of disease.

The purpose of this book is to present to the reader a different paradigm for considering health and disease. The goal is to provide a refocusing of thought toward wellness rather than illness in health care, especially for those who make treatment decisions for children as they grow. The information given here is based on scientific research, as well as on my lifetime of experience as clinician, mother, and grandmother.

First, we will explore factors that shape a healthy life. Then, after taking a look at the systems of the body and how they function together, we'll begin to look at what can go wrong to result in illness. In my next book (*What's Wrong With Me?*) we'll discuss illness processes in more detail, taking a closer look at some non-invasive ways to assist in bringing systems toward a healthier balance. It is my hope that the reader will be left with an appreciation for interventions that truly promote optimal health, along with an understanding that the usual "symptom-relief-with-a-pill" approach of our modern times is not the only option available.

6 6 6

In all stages of life there are factors that influence health and vitality for good or ill. The phrase "use it or lose it" applies to the proper functioning of every system in the body. Learning how to survive *and thrive* in the world outside mother's womb means using and developing *all* systems. Just as

CHAPTER ONE

babies long to kick and stretch and move to strengthen muscles and bones, so too the unseen systems (like the immune system) must learn to identify and overcome the internal and external invaders ever present in our environment. Therefore, paradoxical as it sounds, sickness is an integral part of good health.

A striking development in the overall health picture of Western populations during the last 20 years has been a shift from "bug"-type (infectious) diseases (bacteria, viruses, or microbes causing a sickness) to "metabolic" diseases. Metabolic illnesses are conditions in which the functioning of one or more of the body's systems is compromised. For example, asthma is inadequate lung function, diabetes is the faulty regulation of sugars in the body, and allergy is an overreaction to a normally harmless substance.

The biggest factor in the shift away from infectious disease has probably been dramatic improvement in sanitation (although many attempt to credit vaccination), while one of the major factors contributing to the shift toward metabolic disease has been stress. Causes of increased stress in general include increased use of pharmaceutical intervention for illness, too much technological intervention in the birth process, and very early, very potent immunization schedules.

Stress is something all of us come in contact with every day, but quantifying or comparing different kinds of stress is a tricky business. Factors increasing daily stress levels include too little sleep; chemicals in food, water, and environment; major stage-of-life challenges like school entry, puberty, or a grandparent's death; parents divorcing; and, of course, fears and worry about almost anything. When your stomach rumbles with hunger, it is that stress that makes you start looking for lunch. When you feel cold and put on warmer clothing, stress is the motivator.

Stress, then, has a two-part function: to increasingly *create discomfort* of one sort or another until awareness *prompts action* to relieve the stress and turn off the signals.

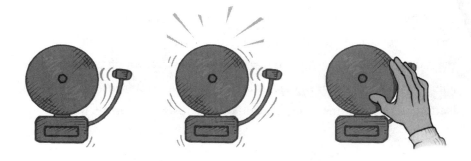

We attend to stress almost continually. For example: Crying baby . . . change nappy (diaper) . . . feed . . . burp . . . back to sleep. Stress signals a need, need prompts a response, response quiets the stress. Sometimes all that is needed is reassurance or a hug, especially if the stress is a bad dream in the middle of the night. We all have different levels that say "enough is enough," and usually we're well aware when that line is crossed. Mild annoyance escalates to action to stop the irritation.

But what happens if the stress is continuous and not relieved time after time? What if stress and fear, which have been shown to produce damaging internal toxins, build up and are not cleared? A build-up of stress-related chemicals affects our nerve and hormone levels, which in turn can alter the functions of virtually every system in the body. When this happens, symptoms of illness often develop, and can include:

- Restlessness
- Irritability
- Poor concentration
- Sleep disturbance, anxiety, depression
- Headache, muscle pain
- Inflammation
- Chronic pain
- Any worsening of a health condition.

CHAPTER ONE

When no intervention occurs to rebalance human stress, a "feedback" loop can develop, with illness causing more stress. For example, allergic reactions can put the body into a very stressed state, which can worsen the allergic reaction. Stomach discomfort or pain can result in a poor diet, leading to nutrient insufficiency and other subsequent problems.

> **In traditional Chinese medicine, symptoms are compared to the branches of a tree, and causes are compared to the roots. For the patient to regain health, both symptoms and causes must be understood and corrected.**

The vast majority of Western literature on health care focuses on illness. In the chapters that follow we will take a different approach, meeting healthy children first. Then we will identify factors that contribute to the growth and development of a child with strong systems. Using positive strategies and making informed choices will provide the best basis possible for any child to achieve a lifetime of optimal health and well-being.

2

Happy, Healthy Children

WHAT DOES A HAPPY, HEALTHY CHILD LOOK LIKE?

There are qualities in a healthy person, or any living creature, that are unmistakable. The first thing observed is the overall physical appearance. The skin and hair are smooth and clear. The eyes have a certain sparkle, a quality called "glitter" in traditional Chinese medicine that indicates the life force or energy level. The child appears contented yet interested, energetic but calm, and alert to his or her environment. Healthy children are, for the most part, pleasant and cooperative if approached reasonably; they generally feel secure in the company of their parents even when presented with new situations. Such children have a strong drive to master whatever skill they are presently working to develop, and they exhibit persistence within an appropriate timeframe.

The everyday routine of a healthy child is largely predictable and relatively easy once one is familiar with his or her needs and particular ways of communicating those needs. A child's first language is *movement*. Adults soon come to recognise the eye rubbing and ear pulling of a sleepy baby. Thumb sucking or fist sucking can mean hunger or distress in some children. A healthy child is a happy child most of the time. If needs are interpreted correctly and met promptly, child and parents begin an effective (at first unspoken) communication pattern that can make life enjoyable and mutually satisfying. When there is a health problem, even as early as in the newborn period, that problem will have an effect on the child's behaviour and moods. There is no such thing as a "naughty baby," just a baby with a problem that is not yet recognised and resolved.

Parents have the responsibility of caring for their young children physically, emotionally, and spiritually. This responsibility includes making decisions about their health, in addition to teaching them the skills they need in order to learn and progress. Parents also pass on values to their children through their example—for better or for worse.

> **When it comes to children, actions speak much louder than words. To repeat: A child's first language is physical—actions.**

Extended family and friends may be resources to parents and can support with advice and help. Professionals may offer expert opinion that is often timely and just as often replaced by the next theory in a few years. Ultimately, the decisions—and the final responsibility for those decisions concerning their children—rest squarely on the shoulders of the parents.

THE BROKEN DREAM

Australia's international image in the 1970s and 1980s was a place of vast open spaces and lean, tanned, fit individuals both young and old. It arguably offered one of the best lifestyles in the world. This was especially true for families. The country had one of the highest rates of home ownership in the world and offered many forms of social support. In the United States of

HAPPY, HEALTHY CHILDREN

America the image of the suburban dream and the land of opportunity promised achievement limited only by ambition and hard work. Both these nations were looked to by the rest of the world as models of "the good life" for their citizens. They offered a seemingly infinite array of foods, commodities, health care, and technology at affordable prices. They had it all and used it "to the max."

By extension, the logical assumption was that the children of this golden lifestyle would grow up happy, healthy, and smart, and live long and well.

The story should go something like this . . .

> Boy meets girl . . .
> They fall in love . . .
> Get married . . .
> Have beautiful babies . . .
> Life is sweet . . .
> Everyone is healthy and happy . . .

Their kids go to school, are eager to learn, to play sports . . . are good at some things, need more practice at others.

This next generation grows up healthy, happy, and sound in mind and body. They are satisfied and grateful for having their choice of unlimited opportunities.

As teenagers they go to college, or learn a trade, or find something they are interested in—something they do well, enjoy, and get paid for doing. Then . . . this boy meets that girl . . . and it starts all over again.

The rest are details and circumstances that make life interesting and challenging.

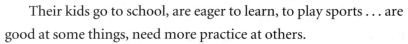

This, then, is:

The American Dream
The Australian Dream

CHAPTER TWO

It's almost the 20th-century version of *It's a Wonderful Life,* that movie classic starring Jimmy Stewart and Donna Reed or, more recently, *The Brady Bunch.* Simple and easy, isn't it?

So why has "The Dream" eluded so many of us?

What happened? Why the broken homes and broken hearts, the drug use and depression among these children of opportunity?

Two generations down the track from "having it all," these two countries have been seeing results that are nigh unto catastrophic for children and their health and happiness.

Australia has one of the highest rates of young male suicide in the world. Drug use among children and teenagers in both countries has escalated to epidemic proportions. Many US children are now grossly overweight, unfit, and drugged for such problems as learning and behaviour disorders, allergy and asthma, attention deficit disorder, and depression. The number of individuals *not* on "medication" is unknown but likely to be small. [Case in point: Bill Rea's attempt to find students at a Texas university who grew up drug-free (pharmaceutical as well as "recreational") to take part in a study failed, and the study had to be cancelled due to lack of a "clean" control group. He just couldn't find enough young people who had not been given significant amounts of drugs.[1]] A few years later, Australian children for the most part followed the same path to the same problems.

ⓑ ⓑ ⓑ

The drug solution has not worked well for many. The consumerism "solution" has not led to contentment either. And throwing vast amounts of money at these problems hasn't made them go away.

Parents are running out of acceptable "expert advice" to resolve the problems their children experience. In most areas of research there is too much information to sift through, with much of it hard to understand and filled with specialized language and conflicting advice.

Everyone loves a quick fix. From the 1950s onward TV scriptwriters brought us heroes who solved the most difficult problems, averted the most horrific disasters, and saved the world from the baddies in one 30-minute episode (with time out for ads). Superman did it, Batman did it, the Lone Ranger did it—*and* left a silver bullet behind to remind us. Nowadays, cartoon action heroes abound and still attempt to save the world from dramatic external threats. Perhaps we are looking in the wrong direction for answers.

If we're really honest with ourselves, most of us go for the easiest solution and, if it doesn't cost too much, all the better. New parents and parents-to-be grapple with choices and pressure to follow this or that method of child rearing. Parents of struggling kids are now in the desperate situation of having to select from a menu of remedies—none of which feels right—just to enable their children to attend school and function at a minimal level.

Parents want their children to grow up healthy, happy, loving, and able to reach their potential and enjoy a satisfying life. However, taking the steps needed to achieve this goal is where the confusion starts. The maze of options is dazzling.

> **It's time to look again at our children and our choices.**

Wherever you are right now reading this book, I want you to stop and look around, then get up and move to another spot. Now you have a new perspective! Same room, different view. This new outlook may allow you to see things that were obscured from view in your last position or maybe allow you some insight into a familiar object in a way that is new and revealing.

Practitioners of traditional Chinese medicine believe that the mind resides within the heart: In order to have peace and health, mind and heart must be in harmony, one with the other.

> **If a solution sounds right to the mind but feels wrong to the heart, it is wise to continue looking until the solution is wholeheartedly acceptable.**

3

Individual Differences

*I*n the same way that no two snowflakes, plants, fingerprints, or puppy dogs are exactly the same, so is each child an individual with characteristics unique to him or her. Even twins who are genetically identical at birth exhibit an infinite variety of distinctive traits.

A TALE OF TWO DONKEYS

Once upon a time, there were two little donkeys plodding along a faraway road. Each was almost hidden under fully loaded baskets. After a time, they came to a river. The donkeys stood on the bank, feeling weary, and sadly gazed across to the other side. The current was swift and the water looked dark and cold.

One donkey carried bags of salt; the other carried baskets full of sponges. The donkey loaded with the salt bags finally spoke. "I shall cross first. At least

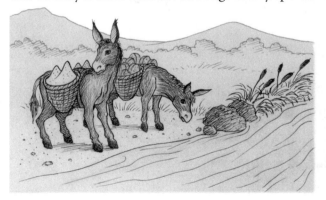

the water will cool me off and wash away some of the dust." He carefully picked his way down among the stones into the river, and soon felt the rising currents swirling around his middle. As water rushed through the bags and dissolved the salt, the little donkey was astonished to feel his burden gradually lessening until it disappeared.

Upon reaching the opposite shore, the relieved donkey called across to his mate still hesitating on the other bank: "It's a miracle, my friend, try it! Just cross the river, and your burden will disappear too."

The second little donkey stepped gingerly into the water, which rose higher and higher over his shoulders, filling the baskets he carried. The sponges, of course, soaked up every drop they could, ultimately causing the hapless donkey—floundering under the increasing weight—to drown.[1]

ⓑ ⓑ ⓑ

What, exactly, is the moral of this little story? Just this: Every individual is unique, and what brings relief to one may be deadly to another.

Children are as different as their billions of genes can make them. Children who may appear to be similar in terms of behaviour and health problems might actually be struggling with completely different underlying issues. Naturally, then, each child requires individual analysis and intervention to resolve his or her problems. Part of the solution may lie in making changes to the daily routine, or to food choices and exercise. Most problems are the result of more than one factor, and so may require a multifaceted solution.

> **Each person has a unique pattern of health and illness.**

If these patterns are identified and specific requirements met, better health becomes achievable. Each person's needs for nutrients, rest, repair, level of activity, and stimulation—essential for that individual's health—will be different (even if only slightly) from every other person's requirements. This fact is a critical one to keep in mind when looking for ways to promote your child's optimal health. Individuality is impossible to cater to when we consider only same-age (or other), large *groups* of individuals.

Ideally we should work vigorously and rest completely in our own natural cycles, tuning in to our bodies' pattern, seasonally and daily.

> **Our biorhythms are the tides of our energy levels.**

A GARDEN OF CHILDREN

A familiar example of diversity among individuals can be found in any garden. Plants can be tiny, or huge, or anything in between. Each type of plant has its individual requirements. Violets prefer a shady spot; fruit trees and roses need lots of sunshine. Some vegetables like potash, but potatoes will grow scabby in it. Cactus needs sand and will rot in heavy, wet clay, even though the soil is rich in nutrients; willows and irises thrive in these soggy conditions and will be stunted in sandy soils.

So plants, trees, and flowers have special individual requirements for nutrients and conditions. When caring for a garden it helps to know which plants need what: when to prune, when to propagate; when to feed, when to water; when to allow periods of rest. Special needs will vary with the seasons of the year. Differences due to specific locations of individual plants—even those of the same type—will lead to different requirements.

> **Knowing what to look for is a key to success.**

Like plants and animals, each person is totally unique. Particular influences will determine a person's needs. These can include season, location, nutritional level, genetic factors, stress, toxic exposure, and bacterial or viral attack. All these influences can vary over time. Again, children are as different as their billions of genes can make them. Differences in development (growth), experiences, perception (the way information is seen and understood), and personal biochemistry all contribute to making each of us truly unique. Every child develops his or her own pattern of responding to challenges. Awareness

CHAPTER THREE

of these individual patterns can make all the difference in applying the correct support when needed.

All plants and children need room to spread out and sink down roots. They need consistent care and guidance. They need sunshine and showers—times of ease and times of challenge, when digging deep for nourishment is required. They need opportunities to give—to share their fruits, and discover the happiness that they alone can create.

Gifts and talents lie latent within each newborn like seeds in a packet. In order to grow and develop, these seeds need to be nurtured and their individual requirements at least partly supplied. Just as each seed in a garden has its own best environment and conditions, so too does each child and each talent. Children learn who they are partly by the reactions and responses they receive from others. All will naturally thrive in an environment of love, support, stimulation, and encouragement. Fortunate is the child who receives thanks for his kindness, support in his challenges, and love for being himself.

If a child's gift is music, what sort of environment would assist the development of that talent? Certainly hearing music would be helpful. Being given time to listen and explore sound and song would be useful. Access to instruments or to tools to *make* simple instruments, and, perhaps, instruction might be supportive.

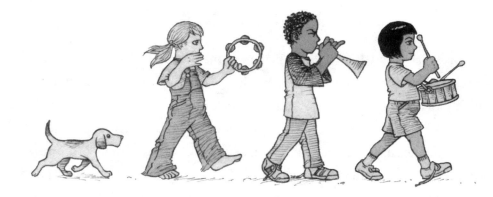

INDIVIDUAL DIFFERENCES

Always the drive to develop talents should come from *within the child*. This intention, this drive to achieve mastery, is the only motivation that will last. The joy and satisfaction needed to sustain the long hours of discipline necessary for realising success can only be generated internally. What constitutes "success" should be defined by the child as well. When a child has accomplished what feels like success, and wants to devote time and attention to some other talent or endeavour, that's the signal to stop and rest, or change tracks.

Presuming that any newborn baby will be just like Mum, Dad, Grandpa, or anyone else is a sure road to unhappiness for all concerned. We've all seen tiny footballs in a two-week-old boy's room, or ballet slippers wrapped up for a new little girl. As parents, we're often tempted to provide children with the means to fulfil those dreams of ours that we never realised—the lost opportunities of the past: the pony, the piano, the dance lessons. But children have their own dreams, and every child deserves the freedom to discover and work toward individual goals without the pressure of having to make Mum's or Dad's come to life too.

> **A mother gives birth. The child chooses a life. A crucial aspect of good parenting is recognising the right time to let go.**

4

Growth and Development: My World

In the first five years of life a child experiences the most rapid rates of learning and growth he or she will ever know. Half (50%) of an entire lifetime of knowledge is accumulated during these years. For such a very young child, the desire to explore is irresistible, and curiosity insatiable. This inner driving force is responsible for the preschooler's incredible speed of development. The importance of this window of opportunity cannot be overemphasized.

The single most beneficial influence in a child's life is having the secure base of an enduring, loving relationship with one person and a cohesive, supportive family unit. Research repeatedly demonstrates that love and consistency in a strong family environment are powerful forces for the development of smart, healthy, resilient children.[1]

Mother provides the child's first environment—her voice, heartbeat, emotional states, food. She represents the safety and security of the baby's entire world before birth, and hopefully during the early years after birth. From this primary experience of love comes the second most important essential for health: love and concern for others.[2] These two facets of love are literally life-savers, because, while the essentials for *life* are air, water, shelter, and nutrients, it is relationships of love and trust that are among the most critical factors for *health*.[3] The quantity, quality, and availability of these life essentials influence growth, repair, and development. These are the basic facts. How they apply to the growing child is the subject of this chapter.

☙ ☙ ☙

The journey from fertilised egg to child-at-school lasts a few short years in time, but represents a leap of light years in terms of development and learning. The milestones of this amazing growth period can be marked in three major areas: physical (or physiological), mental (or cognitive), and emotional (or behavioural).

We could say growth is fastest at conception and gradually winds down over a lifetime. Charting growth and development reveals patterns that are not linear and even; progress is made in bursts and lags. The child often focuses on mastering one task or area of learning almost to the exclusion of all others.

Watching a baby attempting to move from one place to another is a fascinating but frustrating exercise. It seems like so much effort for such negligible gain. However, if we consider this effort in terms of process rather than immediate result, we begin to appreciate the baby as an athlete in training. Just as one could not train for a week and expect to lift a large set of weights correctly and without injury, the baby's "frustrated" movements and energy "randomly" expended are actually very purposeful and precisely tailored for mastering the required task. How many movements it will take for a given child to reach competency is very much an individual and complex matter. It is apparent, though, that learning occurs in spikes or steps rather than smooth curves of continuous progress. The final deep satisfaction of "I did it!" is the best motivator for taking on the next challenge.

Child development may be seen from a variety of perspectives. The child health nurse is looking for measurements within an *average* range: height, weight, head circumference, hearing, vision. Parents are interested in a good night's sleep and a peaceful household. Teachers are looking for the ability to learn and remember new information and skills. Family and friends want the new child to fit into their social structure and learn to behave in certain ways. As long as all internal systems are operating well, a child is open to learning any or all of these various tasks.

To succeed at childhood requires a high degree of functionality and adaptability. Let's look at this challenge from the child's point of view.

From the time of conception, a child inhabits a defined, contained, nurturing space in the mother's body. For the child, the womb is the world. The redefinition ("re-cognition") of this personal world that proceeds day-by-day is the result of a combination of factors. Genetics, environment, personal awareness, and choice, as well as, of course, circumstance all contribute to the individual's development. Therefore, each of us begins life with a personal history (handbook) and challenges (roadmap), which unfold in unique cycles of ups and downs. We require learning and growth to keep making progress. One's own particular *process* of growth and learning and adaptation forms a pattern even before birth.

Once the new baby is born, the world expands dramatically to encompass interaction with the mother, who can now be *seen*. Although initially there is no sense of "self," of existence as a separate being, gradually this new world of mother comes to include all the family and places and sensory experiences that baby will know as "home." The child eventually becomes a part of the family and community; others gain access into the private world a little at a time.

Each child has his or her individual space and perception from the very beginning. Right after birth, an infant's visual range of focus corresponds exactly with the distance to the mother's face while resting in her arms. As the baby grows, the visual scope enlarges to include expanding horizons. Picture a boy or girl inside a large dome that encompasses the individual's existence,

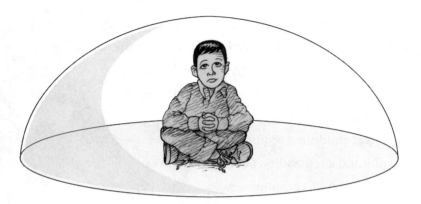

but also protects it, and provides a view. We can call this bubble surrounding the child a Personal Observation Dome (POD). Before birth this enclosure is small and fluid (mother's womb). Throughout life, this space expands or contracts; becomes full and rich, or diminished, broken, and distorted; is polished, tarnished, decorated, or otherwise affected from inside and out. The atmosphere contained in this critical space acts as a filter, influencing interpretation and understanding of both internal and external worlds. In the POD, experiences are processed and either integrated, becoming part of the individual, or stored for future exploration. Experiences can be helpful or difficult, useful or confusing. They can assist and nurture, or present challenges to be overcome.

NATURAL PATTERNS

The processes that support life are not always warm and fuzzy. There is an important natural law called "the adversity principle." Adversity plays a key role in development. It is an essential process for growth. When the chick no longer fits inside the shell and the food supply is just about used up, the chick's inner drive and intuitive knowledge tell it to start pecking. If the chick is assisted in its struggle for life, it does not develop the strength needed to survive, and it usually dies. What appears at first to be a kindness (helping it break out of the shell) is really interference and, ultimately, a death sentence.

Natural processes have determined the most successful strategies for maintenance through growth and development; interference with these may have costly consequences.

Of course, the stress of birth is the first dramatic challenge we all naturally experience. The sudden and cold entry into a new world outside the mother is the final trigger that stimulates a full-on stress response in the newborn. All systems are primed in this way to begin intensive learning. In that first hour, triggers, responses, and imprinting are happening at incredible speed. Sucking, recognising mother, and breathing air must all be learned quickly in order to survive … nature prepares the newborn to be on full alert, to take it all in and learn rapidly, through the challenge of stress. An infant who has not been able to gather up all available resources under the influence of this stress response may be low in muscle tone, slow to breathe, slow to suck—may be generally non-reactive. Often, a Caesarean birth or the use of drugs can compromise the infant's essential responses.[4]

We tend to think that growth occurs mainly in childhood, slowing down and then reversing in older age—becoming degeneration. If we look more closely at growth and repair, we see that these are processes that maintain all living organisms, including you and me, throughout our lives. Growth is simply more noticeable in childhood because of the speed at which it happens. We all grow, for better or worse, until we die. Our bodies are in a continual state of repair. We fix damage in tissues and organs by making new cells. At the same time we get rid of waste products and break down, then eliminate, broken dead cells.

In his book *Unweaving the Rainbow*,[5] Richard Dawkins explains the mystery of appearances. It is a useful analogy for understanding that, although the physical body *appears* solid, we are actually in a state of constant change.

A rainbow appears fixed, but it is actually a *sequence* of water droplets *passing through* a ray of light. As one drop falls, another takes its place, refracting the light in a seemingly unbroken band of colour to the eye of the observer. The viewer sees the rainbow as a unique display. If one moves to a different vantage point one sees a *different* rainbow at the new location.

During every second of our lives we are continuously discarding and replacing cells, just like the water droplets that move through a rainbow. Therefore, like a rainbow, we are never the same at any two moments in time.

These realisations can help us see our bodies as the complex and constantly changing systems they are. Repair and growth are processes inherent in living organisms or systems. Interventions to support or improve upon these processes can be a viable choice at any time in a person's life.

Think of the effect of changing seasons on a tree in a garden or in the woods. Although it comes to life in springtime and is in the exact same location as last year, a series of photos over time would highlight obvious changes which take place through new growth. Its overall appearance, size, and shape would vary from year to year because of differences in the colours of leaves, and changes in the number of branches. New growth is governed by climate, rainfall, nutrients in the soil, location in the garden, sunlight, and how well the tree's other requirements are met during that particular season.

Think of a favourite beach or section of ocean. The ocean tides rise and fall to roughly the same levels, but the seawater itself, the shells and debris washed up onto the shore, and the fish and creatures that are brought in from the depths are all different in every tide.

EARLY DEVELOPMENT

The human child has the longest period of dependency of all the species on earth. The complexity of life skills required for human children to survive on their own necessitates this extended apprenticeship. There have been so many theories about child development that it is difficult to settle on a single viewpoint.

Children's development is, generally speaking, of two types. The first type is readily observable, and can be seen, measured, and recorded. Indicators of this type of growth include height, weight, head circumference, and other measures. External physical development is obvious.

The second type of development is more subtle and can only be observed indirectly. Its unseen master controls are the internal metabolic processes, which themselves are regulated by what can be called "innate intelligence." As an example, consider the fact that once a baby is born and begins breathing, he or she doesn't need to be coached every day to get better at it. Internal drives and metabolic controls kick in and take over. Oxygen inhaled allows cells to grow and operate. The result is the overall growth we can see.

>   internal intelligence
> + metabolic processes
> = growth

The visible (the seen) and the invisible (the unseen) work together to achieve the balance we call growth. It is changing every second, but it is regulated, balanced, and directed by the innate intelligence of each cell. The harmony of growth is simply breathtaking.

The brain comprises a very large percentage of the infant's entire being. It stands to reason that the brain will do most of the organisation and learning needed for survival. Each child must gain knowledge of the world, and in a sense create an individual guidebook for life. The infant gains this knowledge at first through muscle movement. We have all noticed how much a new baby moves—fist, tongue, facial expressions, kicks, and stretches. First we experiment and learn the outcome; then we repeat the experiment, putting in the required practice; then, finally, we achieve our goal. Eventually exploratory movements become deliberate and directed—grasping, smiling, and rolling over have been learned. This is the observable pattern throughout early childhood.

For the first four to five years the child is structuring brain patterns from *sensory experiences*. The nature of this early learning has, almost exclusively, to do with physical mastery and the laws of the real world. Think of a toddler learning to crawl and then walk. Watch a small child eat and drink. A listing of the laws of physics used to accomplish even simple tasks mastered by the child would be a book in itself. This knowledge base, acquired through exploration and experimentation, is the basis of all future learning, leading up to the crowning achievement of conceptual abstract thinking, usually occurring from age 10 or 11 onward. The more safe access a child has to the natural world for learning firsthand through direct contact, the more extensive will be that child's knowledge structure.

How are basic needs for growth and development met in our modern society? Let's review the main tasks of the child.

> **The task of the child in the first four to five years is to structure brain patterns from sensory experience.**

- *Task*: Manipulate the physical environment to experiment and create.

- *Task*: Explore and master movement, language, manipulation, social skills, the physical world.

- *Task*: Map and interact with the real world and the plants and animals and people who share it.

GROWTH AND DEVELOPMENT: MY WORLD

Full development of a child's intelligence requires real-life experiences, not plush toys or mechanical games. When we observe the products offered for babies and small children that supposedly contribute to their growth there are very few which encourage interaction with the real world. If we apply the standards of *primary sensory experience with the natural world* and *the ability to create, invent, and manipulate objects into multiple use tools*, we can see how the toy market falls far short of enhancing learning and development.

- Plastics
- Electronic pictures (TV, computer)
- Restriction for long periods of time (playpens, car seats)
- Artificial, sterile environments
- Structured, complete toys which prevent invention

It is often observed after Christmas celebrations or a birthday party that small children will spend more time playing with the boxes and wrappings than the toys. These offer scope for imagination and creativity, which the single-purpose toy did not.

When we look at the human child we find an ordered pattern of growth, but there is also an unstructured element that will be developed by a particular child in a unique family and set of circumstances. Children participate in their own development through individual choices and perceptions. If opportunities to choose and experience firsthand are absent, if everything is pre-organised and sterilised, growth and development are stifled.

Even if your experience with gardening is quite limited, I'm sure you've noticed the enormous diversity of plants on this beautiful planet. They range from the minute mosses and lichen to the giant redwood standing 300 feet tall and living for centuries. Natural living environments are essential for the development of basic structural learning foundations. These environments can be as tiny as an ants' nest under the cement or as big as a farm or a forest. People are living systems, not computers for storing information and facts.

CHAPTER FOUR

Facts and formulae are best gathered from primary sources: observation and experimentation with the real world. Hands-on experience with the natural world is the most effective classroom.

An observed experience in a preschool in Connecticut which my daughter attended illustrates these points. As the four-year-olds arrived one at a time, they were greeted and encouraged to explore the space where they would spend the morning. The squeals of delight as discoveries were made will always be my definition of learning. A box of real bunnies uncovered in a corner, a half-built cubby-house, and other child-friendly materials waiting to be worked on in other areas all became food for grand imaginations in tiny bodies. The environment was appropriate and safe; it encouraged exploration, experimentation, and creativity. There were adults (teachers) in the room to support and assist, but they were clearly a resource, not directors of the morning's activity.

That classroom was a reflection of the natural world around us. There is an order underlying all growth and all of life's processes. Seeds sprout in a predictable manner to produce an organism that is recognisable, growing in a certain way to a certain height. This new, adult plant, in its natural state, will produce a flower, a fruit, and ultimately a seed—which, when placed in moist soil, will produce yet another member of the same species. This order is seen in all aspects of the natural world. However, there is also randomness, or disorder. Creativity is preceded by access to raw materials in an unordered state, better known as chaos.[6]

> **Everything has its opposite.**
> **Life proceeds in cycles of birth and death.**

The balance of winter and summer is needed for plants and animals that have adapted to seasonal climates. The balance of order and freedom is needed for full realisation of growth potential.

ENHANCING DEVELOPMENT: STAGES

The passage through stages or cycles can be challenging, exhilarating, painful, or sometimes all of these at once. Life is a progression. Change is part of every day, and continues throughout a lifetime. It is not a process unique to childhood. An attempt to stop the growth process at any stage—baby, age 18, 21, 40, 60—will be an exercise in conflict.

Seeing the same world at different ages in life reflects the changes: a child runs for the swings; a grandfather looks for the bench and any dangers.

It has been said that the only constant is change. Our attitude of acceptance, or of resistance, to change can make life either a great adventure or a terrifying ride over the edge. You will be a different parent to your third child than you were to your first child, whatever your age or experience. Children dance their own steps, and parents' steps often fit more readily with one than another. It's often from the child with whom we struggle that we learn the most.

We are on a journey together—parent and child—and we need to change in response to inner and outer challenges, just as the world around us is changing. If we don't, we become isolated and disengaged, as have so many of our elderly—and, increasingly, our youth.

One of the most important areas of development is that of character. Attributes such as honesty, helpfulness, resiliency, loyalty, and humour must be nurtured and developed like any other quality.

Growth proceeds in patterns that follow specific timeframes and present certain requirements. Being aware of and meeting needs during the different stages of growth are crucial parenting skills. Children's role models can encourage particular characteristics to emerge and find expression. The values held by significant people in a child's life leave indelible impressions that can help—or hinder—the development of positive character traits.

Core beliefs are passed on to children much more by what is observed than by what is spoken. If there is a conflict between what parents say and what parents do, the stronger message is in the action. Remember—a child's first language is body language and action.

CHAPTER FOUR

For example, if parents use tobacco, or alcohol—even caffeine—as drugs to "pick them up" when tired, or use pharmaceutical drugs to get going, to get to sleep, or to relax, the message passed on is that it's okay to use drugs to feel better. Parents do not get to choose which drugs are okay and which they don't approve. The value passed on is, "Drugs are okay." This is especially true when parents choose to use drugs to modify their *child's* behaviour.

The way a child is dealt with in everyday situations sets up a pattern. Does a daughter experience kindness or harshness, flexibility or rigidity, consistency or chaos, excuses or accountability? Is she acknowledged at all, or does she usually go unnoticed? Early learning is the foundation of a child's character. Of course there are exceptions—a child whose character shines even in the worst of circumstances.

It is extremely important to understand that the child from birth to three years cannot knowingly disobey or wilfully misbehave. When a baby is crying or upset, *there is a reason*. The caregivers involved may not be able to figure out what's wrong, but it is not the baby's intention to spoil a dinner, or upset the family, or keep anyone from getting a good night's sleep. The cry is simply communication in the only language an infant knows.

What do children *really* need during their first five years?

- *Time*: To be alone, to be with parents, with others, with the natural world; unstructured time for creating, thinking, experimenting.

- *Safety*: Both physical and emotional.

- *Love*: Unconditional and consistent.

- *Basic needs*: Food, shelter, water.

- *Freedom* (age appropriate): To explore the natural world, to explore materials for self-expression and creativity.

- *"No"* when appropriate.

- *Parents* who can discern what is too much, too little and "just right" in a given situation through thorough knowledge of their child.[7]

Enhancing the child's development would certainly include responding to individual needs and interests. Knowing when to stand back and recognising when to intervene are equally important. These parenting skills can only be learned by putting in the time and effort to interact with, observe, and form a close relationship with one's child.

⚙ ⚙ ⚙

Human infants travel a long, slow road toward autonomy. Autonomy is the result of knowledge and ability. Abstract thinking in the adult arises from the concrete thinking of the child. Progression toward pure thought is genetically programmed and unfolds in neat, sequential stages. Internal rewards (far superior to external rewards) preserve the driving motivation to master speech, movement, and discovery that is so evident in the early development of a child. Accomplishments are their own satisfaction; no stickers or stamps saying "good boy" or "well done" are needed. The internal "aha!" of discovery, followed by learning, practice, and mastery, is satisfaction enough.

Has anyone "spoiled a surprise" for you by telling you what's in a gift before you've opened it? Or when you gave a handmade gift has the recipient asked you "what is it?"—when "it" just *is*—and to you is *beautiful*? This lack of understanding, comprehension, and empathy creates wariness and distrust, and in fact makes you hesitate to disclose yourself to that person again.

CHAPTER FOUR

An internal reward results from the joy of doing or attempting a task.

An external reward feels more like a judgment, an evaluation of how one's work (and therefore one's self—the creator of that work) measures up to someone else's standard or opinion. In fact, in many areas of practical life and academic achievement, learning and success have been shown to be directly correlated with the number of mistakes made. The manner in which errors or mistakes are dealt with in the learning process can either enhance or negate this valuable tool.

There's a saying in Emergency Services: "You can live three weeks without food, three days without water, and three minutes without air." It gets the priorities right for which compromised essentials must be addressed immediately for *survival*: airway blockage and breathing certainly come first.

Remember, though, that a child's most important essential for *health* is love: nurturing, supportive, unconditional love.

5

Structure and Function

STRUCTURE: THE COMPONENTS OF A SYSTEM

When observing any living thing, what can be seen by the naked eye is only part of the story. If we look at a tree, we see its visible features: trunk, branches, and leaves. We don't see the roots underground. We don't see nutrients flowing upward under the bark. We don't see food being manufactured in the green leaves when the sun is shining. We don't see carbon dioxide entering or oxygen exiting through those leaves.

In fact what we do see—what we can touch and inspect—is probably the simplest part of the tree. No matter how long our observation lasts, and even if we record every detail we notice, we certainly could not say we know everything about it. We have simply seen *part* of its structure. Even after cutting it down, taking measurements, and recording what's inside, we cannot understand how the tree works as a living entity.

Trees, puppy dogs, children, and all living things have *structure*. They also have *function*.

FUNCTION: HOW A SYSTEM WORKS

In addition to observing structure, we can learn about living things by watching how they act, grow, and repair. Observing behaviour gives us valuable information. Even sunflowers, which appear to stay pretty much in one place, do move. They simply move too slowly for the human eye to see (unless you are very patient and spend the entire day with one).

There are many ways to get information about living things. Most of the scientific information we have comes from the study of structure, which has given us answers to questions like: What is it made of? How big is it? What does it look like on the outside? What about on the inside? Scientists have compiled mountains of data about much of the world we live in and the creatures that share the planet with us. We know about the stars, the solar system, and the universe. Physical laws governing the world, and the parts of it that can be seen and measured, have recently been studied and recorded as never before.

Most of the early information about people was gained from the study of corpses (deceased people). Scientists and artists had to perform their experiments in secret because of taboos surrounding death, and much debate arose from the failure to find any physical structure that could be called the human "soul," or "spirit," in a corpse. These early studies of the physical human being have contributed greatly to our knowledge of how the body and organs are formed. Many assumptions about the living made from the study of the dead were later proven wrong. The thymus gland, for example, was believed to be superfluous in adults, because in young soldiers killed in war this gland was shrivelled and useless. We know now that under stress the thymus gland shrinks and "burns out."[1] After recovery, though, it becomes a functioning and useful organ once again, aiding in (among other things) the intricate interplay of internal chemical communication that gives rise to, and is affected by, emotions.[2] In fact, through our thoughts we generate feelings, which then become chemicals in the body *via* secretions of our endocrine glands, which in turn influence how we think. As we'll see, it's a loop that can be broken from the inside as well as the outside.

STRUCTURE AND FUNCTION

The belief that "If you can't see it, then it doesn't exist" has now fallen into disrepute, but not completely without a cost. There is still great reluctance to accept the unseen—that which can't be measured and manipulated.

Health has long been equated with *structural* perfection. A real trend of late is having cosmetic surgery to "roll back the years." Does smooth, wrinkle-free skin actually indicate a healthy system? Yes—and no. If the skin is smooth and wrinkle-free due to excellent nutrition, a healthy lifestyle, and well-functioning internal systems, the answer is yes. If the skin is smooth due to stretching, cutting, and plumping up with collagen (or fat from your bottom), and the systems inside are ancient, clogged with rubbish, and not working very well, the answer is no. Appearances can be deceiving.

More recently, *function* (how well does it work?) has been recognised as the other (perhaps more important) half of the health equation. This second part of the story is best detected indirectly, mainly through behaviour. Function includes growth and efficiency in essential areas like energy production, repair, intelligence, and learning, among many others.

How does a daffodil, which is stored up in a bulb all winter, know when the exact right time to start growing has arrived? Then, when its season is over, how does it tuck its energy and blueprint back into the bulb until next year?

Which really is the daffodil?

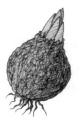

The bulb?

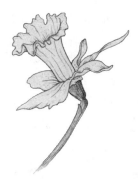

Or the flower?

CHAPTER FIVE

There is an additional dimension in the study of living things that is recently coming into scientific awareness. That dimension is relationship. Albert Einstein had his aha! moment when he discovered that the *relationship* between two or more things is as important (or maybe more important) than the individual things on their own. This is Einstein's theory of relativity in a nutshell. The famous $E=MC^2$. Just about anything will behave differently in a different situation or environment. Even a person.

Think of yourself or your child at home, and then at school or work, and then at a party with peers. It becomes quite obvious that changing one's environment—being with other people in different places—exerts an influence on each of us. Even being alone has its influence.

In our example of trees and plants, we saw how location can have an impact on growth and health. If a particular tree needs rich soil but is growing in sand, that will have a definite effect on its ultimate size and health. We can find other influences of environment—in challenges, care received, and the other inhabitants of that space.

A living being consists of:

- *Structure*: The physical parts.
- *Function*: How those parts interact and work.

and is affected by:

- *Environment*: Influences both good and bad.

In addition, we have to acknowledge a certain "X" factor, which is none of the above. We could call this "life," or "energy," or "spirit." It is about the sum being greater than its parts. If we made a robot that could perform all the functions of a person—even thinking and being somewhat creative (such as a computer playing chess or painting)—that "talented" robot would still be a machine. Even if a robot could mimic all of a human being's *behaviours*, the spark of life, self-determination, and unique personality would still be missing.

Where does a person's *experience* fit into this description of living things? Experience (or perception) can be described as an individual's unique impact on, or understanding of, an event or interaction.

CAR MODEL
Structure

A vehicle has many parts, such as:

- Tyres
- Radiator
- Horn
- Gas tank
- Seats
- Roll bar (chassis)
- Steering wheel
- Brakes
- Fan
- Lights
- Mirrors
- Windows
- Doors

These are the physical structures that to a large extent will determine its best use: truck, limousine, racing car, van, or RV.

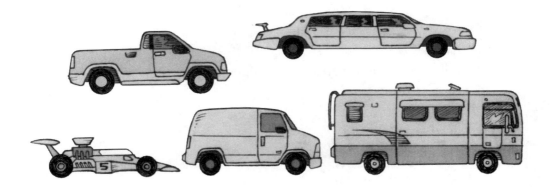

It may be built for speed, for comfort, for hard work, or for fuel economy.

Function

"Function" is defined by how all the parts work together. "Good" function implies that the level of repair required to maintain proper output is reasonable.

CHAPTER FIVE

LIVING THINGS: STRUCTURE *AND* FUNCTION

When we apply this simple car analogy to human health, we see that *structure* refers to any physical part of the body—the organs and tissues; heart, blood, bones, lungs, kidneys. Internal structures of the living body can be seen and described using scans or x-rays.

Function in a living being refers to what an organ does, alone and in conjunction with other organs. Parts and structures overlap and interlace, as do their functions. Some organs and tissues have obvious functions—bones support all our other organs, for example. Others operate in unseen, less obvious, very complex ways. In addition, groups of organs function together in *systems*. Finally, all these systems work in wondrous unity to allow the life-endowed entity to carry out essential tasks.

Therefore, while we may artificially separate the body into parts and pieces, it really does need to be seen as a whole. We all have physical gifts and limitations. Working with our particular structure rather than against it makes life a great deal more enjoyable.

Let's look again at our car analogy. Examples of diminished function in a car can include:

- Flat tyre—air missing
- Flat battery—charge down
- Lost key—can't start the car
- Broken fuel line—won't get very far

You get the picture. Many problems of function have obvious causes that are easily discovered.

But what happens when we run into a trickier problem? Everything *looks* okay. The tests on the motor show spark, yes; fuel in carby, yes; leads connected, yes. Everything should be okay, but it isn't. We're not going

STRUCTURE AND FUNCTION

anywhere—not in this car! Ah, the mysteries of auto electronics, fuel injection, and computer systems.

In the living organism, a situation like this could be compared to metabolic dysfunction, or to a problem of programming or energy—that is, a problem not of structure or readily observed function, but of unseen, less easily understandable function.

To illustrate: I heard a health professional discussing Alzheimer's disease on a radio talk show. She made the distinction between everyday "forgetting" and Alzheimer's disease, which involves memory loss due to a kind of neurological dysfunction in the brain that is not understood. Ordinary forgetfulness (structure = brain, function fundamentally intact) may involve misplacing your keys; a person with Alzheimer's disease may well not know what a key is used for.[3]

Later in this book the organs and tissues of the body will be grouped into four functional systems: nutrition, protection, communication, and detoxification. All of these systems are interrelated, and constantly share information. What needs to happen for maintaining the balance and integrity of all the systems is the good health equation:

> sufficient nutrients and essentials
> \+ good elimination of toxins
> = excellent health, growth, and repair

Everything we do has an effect on every other part of us. We are much more complicated than a "factory line." It's not a matter of, "Oops, there's a breakdown at station D." It's more like, "I can't breathe, so all the other systems are going off, too."

Each of our systems has a structure and a function. These aspects of every system can be influenced by unseen energy factors, and environmental factors, that can vary from person to person, from moment to moment.

CHAPTER FIVE

For example, one girl falls out of a tree and breaks her arm. She has it set. The arm heals and is no longer a problem. The girl still climbs trees (a bit more carefully now); structural and functional damage has been repaired.

Another girl falls out of the same tree, breaking her arm. She is traumatized by the ordeal and becomes fearful and stressed. Her arm bone knits and heals, but her fears do not. Her function is impaired. This becomes progressively more of a problem. Not only does she refuse to be adventuresome and climb trees again, she becomes more and more reticent about going anywhere. She clings to home and mother; eventually her problem really doesn't have much to do with the original broken bone. Her fears have a gradual but debilitating effect on growth and development. Appetite decreases, lack of exercise and fresh air affects her systems' abilities to function, and a steady stream of stress hormones begins to stunt her physical, cognitive, and emotional behaviour and development.

Why did one child respond well to treatment and support, while the other did not? There are many factors involved in the answer to that question. For now, it is enough to recognise that while maintaining structure and function within a certain range is necessary for health, these are not the only factors that play a role in wellness and illness. It is through exploring intangible factors (such as relationships, support, role models, love, nurture, affirmation, experience, and understanding) that many answers to today's health issues may be found.

Choosing purely scientific or purely artistic explanations of life (by separating mind from heart) has resulted in two artificial and limited systems of thought. Neither is wholly successful without the other. As with the legendary feud between the McCoys and the Hatfields, the time has come to bury the hatchet, to usher in a new era of cooperation and collaboration between the sciences and the arts. Such a venture, if done in the spirit of discovery and mutual respect, can only result in benefits for all.

STRUCTURE AND FUNCTION

We are dual beings: of matter and spirit (or energy, if you prefer that word), of analysis and creativity—different types of thought processes occurring in the left and right hemispheres of our brains. We need to incorporate aspects of thinking *and* feeling in order to lead truly healthy lives.

6

Too Much, Too Little

A STORY

There once were two children who lived near the sea.

The little boy and little girl were best friends who spent most of their free time playing and exploring on the shore. On sunny days they collected pebbles and seashells that peeked out of the sparkling white sand. On stormy days they looked for scary bits of seaweed and stranded creatures. Once they found a dead seagull and a sea cucumber (it was still alive) and lots of spiky sea urchins. They knew better than to touch the poisonous puffer fish. Yes, the beach was their favourite place to explore.

As the children grew older they decided to collect their favourite sea-things. Almost every day they went on a "treasure hunt" and brought home something to help them remember . . . a "souvenir." They labelled their finds with little white tags, including both the English and Latin names (when they could find them). As time went by, tables in both homes became piled high with "treasure." All their drawers got filled up, then sea-things found their gritty way to every part of both houses: onto the chairs—ouch!—and the beds—double ouch!! Eventually there was hardly room to sit or walk—even into the kitchen—without crunching a favourite bit of coral or seashell.

As time went on, the two friends began to quarrel over their treasures as they became lost or damaged. They sorted and rearranged the piles, growing more and more pale, cranky, and unhappy. Trips to the seashore were rare now.

CHAPTER SIX

One very bright morning they awoke to see a ship sailing on the horizon. They met while running down toward the surf to get a better view. Suddenly they realised how wonderful the sea breeze felt in their hair, and how good the salt air smelled. The sun warmed their shoulders—the sky was a perfect blue. "Why are we spending the summer indoors when we can run and play and explore out here?" they wondered.

Returning home at the end of that wonderful day, the children boxed and bagged all their old "finds." They lugged the whole lot down to the beach (where it all belonged, anyway) and watched as the waves reclaimed the sea's treasure.

The children made a promise that from now on they would be doers, not collectors, treasuring their memories—and each other. They grew strong and healthy out in the fresh, clean ocean air, running and digging and playing and just being . . . children.[1]

> **We often hear the statement:**
> **"You can't get too much of a good thing."**
> **Oh, yes you can. More is not always better, just more.**
> **Sometimes less is better; often — *much* better.**

One of the essentials of life is water. Our bodies are actually 80% water. But, drinking too little water can contribute to diseases such as arthritis, kidney problems, and skin problems.[2] Get too much water in your lungs and you'll drown.

Which would you rather have?

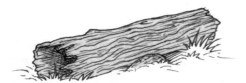 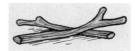

To start a fire at camp: a big log or small twigs?

TOO MUCH, TOO LITTLE

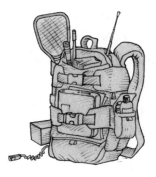
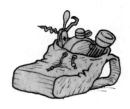

To carry on a short hike: a 50-pound backpack full of everything, or a small rucksack with just the essentials?

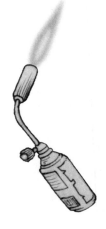

To light a gas stove: a blowtorch or a box of matches?

Bigger is not necessarily better; often *less* is better.

Keeping up with new products and technology has its cost. I know many people over the age of 50 who need a young teen to set their digital watch, to program their VCR, and to guide them through the mysteries of using computers. It can easily take more time to research, select, and buy a replacement electronic item (a faster and more complicated computer, for example) than the time that the new, improved product promises to save. Often what we really need is not a newer, faster, bigger, "You Beaut" widget, but the *time* to use the familiar goods we already have.

CHAPTER SIX

How many of us actually use all of the features on the computers, communication systems, and sound equipment we have now? How many of us go to the upper limits of our car's speed? When would it ever be wise to do so? Why, then, pay for all that "power"?

There is a very useful concept called "the Goldilocks principle." Do you remember the little girl who wandered into the bear's house in the woods? She was lost and tired and hungry. And fussy! One chair was too big, another too little . . . and then she found the one that was just right. She did the same with bowls of porridge on the table: one was too hot, one was too cold. One was just right . . . and she gobbled it up. We can call this idea "too much, too little, and just right." This simple yardstick can serve as a valuable tool to help find the best solutions for very different situations.

When applying the concept to making choices for health, we find that there will be a "best range" in almost every area. Thinking of too much, too little, and just right will help in deciding about food and water intake, amounts of exercise and sleep, or limits on TV and video game time. Making choices within these ranges will result in improved health and happier children (and parents).

The following short story makes the point.

> A new office worker was standing in front of the shredder holding a piece of paper in his hand. A senior secretary walked by.
>
> The new employee asked, "How do you turn this thing on?"
>
> "Here," the secretary said, taking the piece of paper and inserting it into the shredder.
>
> "And where does the copy come out?"

Too little information—too much intervention.

6 6 6

A person whose needs are met can encounter great challenges without being overwhelmed or severely affected (negatively) by those challenges.

The key is that they have achieved and are maintaining their "dynamic balance." This concept can be illustrated in the chemistry laboratory. We see it at work in solutions of liquids. When one adds a salt to a liquid, the salt crystals will begin to dissolve until a certain concentration is reached. If more salt is added at this point, instead of dissolving it will start to settle out in the bottom of the container in the form of crystals. This "saturation point" will differ depending on the type of liquid, its temperature, and the type of salt used, but the process remains the same. Too little salt—it's not at maximum concentration; too much salt—it's oversaturated and begins to settle out; but with the "just right" amount of salt, we have a solution in perfect "dynamic balance."

Let's apply the ideas of "too much . . . too little . . . and dynamic balance" to the questions of exercise and work. When the amount of intense focus, concentration, or mental work exceeds a certain point, one's system goes out of balance. Most people have experienced this; eyes begin to tire, the brain slows, and the body aches from being in one position for too long. At this point, the balance of all one's systems is under strain, and efficiency suffers. (Very like driving a car uphill in fourth gear instead of second.) The strain begins to cause wear and tear.

(In traditional Chinese medicine, the concept of "balance of energy" is important. The situation above would be called "excessive" mental activity, or "overwork," and is thought to create a variety of imbalances that can lead to disease states.)

A better way to work or exercise is to stop frequently for a brief rest, or to do something different for a little while (maybe take a short walk), in order to regain balance. In the case of overuse of mental faculties, some physical activity will restore balance and energy. In the case of physical overuse, water, rest, and mild food will restore balance.

Deepak Chopra, in his book *Perfect Weight*,[3] speaks of an Ayurvedic physician recommending physical exercise as beneficial for body and mind. This physician cautioned that too much exercise could be as harmful as too little. In Eastern medicine and philosophy, mind and body are not thought of separately, but as a single unit. To be useful, it is felt that any practice should benefit the entire being.

Exercise is important for old and young. Children should be encouraged to spend time enjoying physical activities outdoors. However, consider the stress and pressure of Little League competition. In fact, consider the young hopefuls in any competitive endeavour. For every winner there are necessarily dozens of disappointed youngsters. Do these get labelled "losers" (by themselves or others)? Does the pressure of the competition outweigh the benefits of the exercise? Is there another physical activity that might be more enjoyable without the competition?

Excessive physical training can lead to a higher incidence of hypertension, arthritis, and heart disease.[4] Some countries in Eastern Europe have instituted de-conditioning programs for their athletes.[5] In America, the life expectancy of a professional football player is around the late fifties, as compared with the average American's late seventies.[6] When players push themselves past the point where they could happily stop and have a rest—beyond the time when their body says, "It's time for a break"—and continue to play even harder, they begin to dip into reserves of energy and nutrients, and even start to use their own muscle tissue as fuel.[7] This is a classic illustration of "too much." After reserves are depleted, it takes much longer to repair damage and regain former levels of health and vitality.

The reason for this can be simply stated as the principle of balance.

Balance = not too much, not too little = just right

How much more sensible it would be to stop, when the body or mind *says* "stop," to rest for a time, allow repair to take place, then go ahead with activities. It has become a modern virtue to "soldier on," to just keep going and "don't let the team down." In business, the mantra has become "whatever it takes," setting up the expectation that employees will work much too long and hard for the proper maintenance of balance and good health to be a realistic possibility.

We are each different in many ways, and because of those intrinsic differences one formula, or one size, does not, and never will, fit all. The "just right" solution is one we must discover for ourselves. The first step in that process is learning to acknowledge how and what we are feeling. After that, we need to be willing to act accordingly, instead of constantly complying with the "keep going till you drop" culture, then expecting medical technology to make up the difference.

Strengthening ourselves to meet any challenges that are necessary or unavoidable should be part of everyday self-care. Our choices should be made in the light of self-knowledge. Strengths, weaknesses, and situations change.

GOOD	Good nutritional status
HEALTH	+ good detox ability
FORMULA:	= no reaction

This formula was the basis for most medicine in the East and West until about 200 years ago.[8] Faulty elimination of toxins was seen to be the cause of disease. This formula is clearly still important today. It illustrates the principle of balance. It is fundamental as a basic health concept where there is degenerative illness of any kind. Achieving and maintaining vibrant good health affords the greatest protection at any age.

If damaging chemicals, toxins, or substances encountered in daily living are neutralised and eliminated before they can affect the system, we have a non-event. In fact, this process of "detoxing" goes on constantly, throughout our lives, day and night, without a single conscious thought. Maintaining nutrition (with proper diet and support to maximize absorption of essential nutrients) as well as the ability to detox spent byproducts of metabolism are essential functions of life.

Absorption and bioavailability are two major factors frequently overlooked when considering nutrition. A person may swallow ten vitamin pills after breakfast; depending on the ability of the digestive system to absorb the nutrients and their subsequent access to the insides of pertinent cells (bioavailability), they may do some good, or they may be a total waste of money and effort.

> **The effectiveness of our absorption and detox functions is what determines the quality of our health.**

Many people are very conscientious about taking vitamins these days. It is, in fact, a multi-billion-dollar industry. Advertising, which only sometimes includes scientific research, greatly influences most people's choice.

When considering taking supplements or remedies, like this vitamin pill or that herbal formula, there is no solution that will be right for everyone. The only thing of importance is deciding what is needed now, for this person. Again, the idea of ranges or tolerances is a key concept that can be helpful in understanding the role of nutrition in health.

Most nutrients and medications will work best when administered in *context:* what is needed at this time, in this individual, in this situation.

CASE STUDY

Mike is a nine-year-old whose life has been miserable due to chronic allergy. Since the age of three he has been on and off a variety of pharmaceutical medicines for severe hayfever. His symptoms have included a permanently blocked nose, very itchy eyes, and sneezing. He has had numerous medical tests, but no interventions have corrected the problem.

When I saw him, he seemed a very unhappy little boy. He had symptoms of stress, allergy, and low detox function. I used a three-fold treatment approach, based on the principles of Functional Medicine:

- Stress release and energy balance[9]
- Homoeopathic medication (desensitisation)
- Children's herbs for nerve and respiratory function

Mike cooperated fully with taking his herbal medicine and going a bit easier with sports. Three and a half weeks later, Mike and his mother reported complete resolution of the allergy problem. Their comment was: "Wonderful!"

What happened? Balance was regained; after desensitisation to allergens and "just right" herbal support, function improved. In other words, decrease the reaction to allergens (which was "too much"); increase the detox function ("too little" elimination); and, once balanced, keep challenges within a manageable range.

Mike has been more active, with more energy and less reactivity, because he has reserves of nutrients and energy; he chooses foods wisely, keeps up water intake, and doesn't overdo it. He does not need ongoing intervention because he is "just right" (has achieved "balance"). He can now handle the occasional challenge, as long as he stays in his "healthy range."

CASE STUDY

A healthy child, Mary, is exposed to a lawn "weed 'n feed" pesticide-fertiliser combination while playing at her friend's house after school. This exposure had no noticeable effect at the time. Remember the good health formula?

> Good nutritional status
> + good detox ability
> = no reaction

Now let's see what happens when Mary has a cold and has lost her appetite. After eating very little for a whole day, she is exposed to the same chemicals. This time Mary has a mild-to-moderate reaction. She has trouble breathing, gets an all-over rash, and turns a bit orange (liver-ish) around the eyes. The formula now reads:

> Low nutritional status
> \+ high immune activity
> \+ low detox
> \+ exposure
> = reaction

What was easily detoxed *last* week became, on *that* particular day in *that* child's life, a problem of overload, causing a reaction. "Too much, too little" is why sometimes one type of food or pollen will cause sneezes and a runny nose, while at other times the same (or even worse) exposure will not.[10]

CASE STUDY

Sarah is a healthy child—age five years. All her systems are in the healthy functional range on this day—Sarah is feeling well and active. She is provided with:

- Good clean water
- Food
- Rest
- Exercise
- Hugs and cuddles
- Challenges
- Learning
- Social interactions

Sarah is accidentally exposed to chemicals (enamel-based paint) just after having a good, nutritious lunch. She is able to neutralise these chemicals by supporting a vigorous detox process. No problem occurs.

A few weeks later . . . Sarah didn't sleep well because of a cold last night. She's been off her food for a day or two—so nutrient levels are down. She comes into contact with the same chemicals, in the same quantities, in the same place (school), but this time, Sarah's detox mechanisms are on overload getting rid of the microbes from her cold (her immune response is hard at work).

The result: Chemicals slip through the detox process and become more concentrated. They circulate throughout the system, triggering a high level reaction/response. Sarah's breathing becomes difficult, she develops a rash and allergy symptoms, nausea, a headache, and is generally a sick little girl. This time, the same exposure is "too much."

The study of health in relation to surroundings is called "Environmental Medicine." We can see that circumstances combine with an individual's health status—hydration, nutrient level, and integrity of all the systems—to make an impact on the outcome of each challenge every day.

- "Too much, too little, just right"
- "The Goldilocks principle"
- "Dynamic balance"
- "Therapeutic window"
- "Energy balance"

Whatever this concept is called, the truth is the same: In every situation, for every person, there are best practices that lead to health.

There are also unwise choices: poor eating habits, physical overuse, and mental overwork (to name a few), leading to burnout and ill health. It seems obvious that much of the sadness and tragedy in today's culture is the result of exhausted, stressed individuals making poor choices under pressure, often in desperate circumstances.

But evaluating our own "just right" for any given time and situation—the definition of "good health"—should be our priority.

> **Awareness is the first step toward change. Choices made with knowledge give us the freedom to build health.**

7

Assessment

A health assessment is a process used by healthcare practitioners to document changes in growth, function, and development. This results in a description of the current condition of a person's health, which should include an understanding of his or her present level of performance. Recording progress in physical growth is only one part of assessing a child's development.

Assessments are done for many different reasons. The form a given assessment takes depends on what characteristics are being evaluated, who is doing the assessing, and what tools or methods are used to take measurements. Often when an assessment is used to evaluate some aspect of performance, measures taken are compared with standard, or average, degrees of competence. For example, taking a driver's licensing test should provide an assessment of the applicant's qualifications to drive a certain type of vehicle (car, truck, motorcycle, bus); skills evaluated need to include knowledge of street signs and road rules, ability to park or stay on the road (as appropriate), and safety awareness, to name a few. There are minimum standards that must be met before a person is permitted to operate a vehicle on public roads. There are also requirements for periodic re-testing or other evaluations of ongoing performance. If someone accrues a certain number of demerit points, there are consequences that sometimes can be as severe as the loss of driving privileges.

CHAPTER SEVEN

Assessment of driving ability occurs mainly in the areas of knowledge and practical skill; the *applicant's* performance is measured. Another issue pertinent to highway safety, though, is the *vehicle's* performance. If a vehicle is unsafe, it is deregistered and banned from the public road system, even though its owner may be a competent driver. When a car has been "off the road" due to faults in structure or function, it must "go over the pits" for an inspection, to make sure it is safe and roadworthy enough for re-registration and licensing. This inspection must be done by an experienced mechanic, who examines the vehicle's overall appearance and bodywork, the condition of tyres, motor, brakes, lights, and so forth—the *structural* assessment. An assessment of *function* would include an evaluation of how the car's parts are working, how it starts and runs, how it sounds, any excessive noise (muffler and exhaust system), whether it needs a tune-up. The operation of wipers, lights, the radio, and electronic systems would be checked. Taking the car for a test drive would allow for assessment of shock absorbers, front end and handling, brakes, and pick-up for passing when power is needed—of *performance*. Ideally, the assessor is one who has experience in recognising signs of problems before they become dangerous. The RAC (Royal Automobile Club) in Australia offers an assessment service to prospective car buyers. They provide a written report detailing the overall condition of the vehicle, and identifying any particular areas of concern.

A SAMPLE CAR CHECKLIST

STRUCTURAL
- Tyres
- Bodywork
- Engine
- Parts

FUNCTIONAL
- Wiring
- Ignition
- Fuel injectors
- Electronic systems

ASSESSMENT

PERFORMANCE
- Handling
- Power
- Acceleration
- Steering
- Braking
- Comfort

It is essential to know what to look for before beginning any health assessment. The Online Cambridge Advanced Learner's Dictionary[1] defines health as "the condition of the body and the degree to which it is free from illness, or the state of being well." Assessment of a person's health would include an appraisal of the overall picture of health, well-being, and function. The main areas of assessment in our car analogy were structure, function, and performance. In the healthcare field the most common evaluations are physical examination, weighing and measuring, and pathology testing.

Pathology is "the study of characteristics, causes, and effects of disease, as observed in the structure and function of the body."[2] Specific tests can be performed to determine the presence or absence of "pathogens," which are harmful microorganisms ("bugs") capable of producing disease. Tests can also show the presence or absence of functional markers (such as red and white blood cells, or enzymes) which can indicate how well or poorly specific systems are performing.

At times, a child will be growing, and no pathology can be identified, but instinct and observation tell you that "something is not right." This is actually one of the most reliable indicators of illness that we have. Parental concerns and their intimate knowledge of the child are valuable tools in assessing health. Health and happiness are usually companions. When a person feels well, he or she is typically patient and well-disposed toward others. The opposite is often true as well: When a child feels unwell he or she can be difficult, sulky, and uncooperative.

CHAPTER SEVEN

In the absence of any disease or pathology, there is a broad grey area of "... but I just don't feel right, Mummy." Some indicators that all is not well can be "school tummy," anxiety, loss of appetite, aggression, tears. You notice that the sparkle is gone from your daughter's eye. She is quiet when usually a chatterbox. Her appearance is somehow different. These are all signs that something is amiss—but it may not be a "bug" or a broken arm. The problem may lie in the area of emotions, stress, feelings—often in the realm of "too much, too little"—and the result is lowered function.

There are ways of assessing these subtle symptoms of "energy imbalance" using age-old, time-tested tools that rely on observation and experience. They come from the fundamental principles of traditional Chinese medicine, and the more recent fields of Functional Medicine and Behavioural Medicine. They can be used when there is no obvious injury or known serious illness causing the symptoms—situations which should, of course, be addressed immediately.

There are many ways to test energy. One way, which is simple, non-invasive, and accurate, involves testing levels of energy in the meridians, and is done by practitioners of kinesiology. Most people would be able to learn a simple "energy test" in a relatively short time. Dr. Y. Omura has patented his method, which he calls "Bi-Digital O-Ring testing."[3] This method compares strength in the fingers with a particular substance. The reaction can be quite strong, neutral, or very weak. There are also bioresonance machines that will give an energy profile in graph form before and after any treatment.[4] The theory that provides the reasoning behind all these testing procedures is this: The balance of meridians and energy fields is a good indication of overall health.[5]

For many healthcare practitioners, identifying areas of low energy is a valuable aid in selecting possible measures that need to be taken to correct the imbalance. Interventions like these are what preventive medicine is all about. Treating a *potential* source of crippling dysfunction is easier, less expensive, and more rewarding than waiting until the serious condition develops, and only then trying to intervene.

> **Happiness is more than the absence of sadness.**
> **Health is so much more than the absence of disease.**

8

Systems Overview

It is easy to compare the body to any number of mechanical models: a car, a computer, a castle. At times these analogies are very helpful in understanding new information. It is important, however, to keep in mind the complexity of the human being as a masterpiece of creation. There is nothing that even vaguely approaches the organisation and intricacy that is a human infant. I address this subject with a deep sense of reverence and awe. I offer my insights with the realisation that our collective knowledge, extensive though it seems at times, is still very much in its infancy. As research uncovers more and more intricate details of the way our bodies work, it is clear that each system is intertwined with and dependent on every other system—if not literally in a physical, structural sense, then certainly in terms of function.

Sometimes the sheer volume of information on a topic such as children's health is so overwhelming that it seems impossible to take it all in, and we end up "leaving it to the experts." However, as I've stated before and cannot emphasize enough, a child's parents are usually the first to know if something is "not quite right." They may not be able to put a name to it, but whether or not their hunch is confirmed by an "expert," this "gut feeling" is still the most reliable indicator of a problem. As a parent, you need to trust yourself. Your feelings and detailed knowledge make *you* the *true* expert where *your* child is concerned.

CHAPTER EIGHT

This chapter is a very basic primer on how the major systems of the body work together. All the systems that make up a person cannot really be separated one from another. They are interrelated and act as a whole. If one part of the body is not working well (let's use the lungs as an example), the effects (of low levels of oxygen and poor cleansing of carbon dioxide, in this case) will be felt in every cell. However, in the interest of simplicity, we will first briefly focus on one system at a time, and then take a look at how they interact and rely on each other in everyday life.

For the purposes of this book the organs and tissues of the body will be grouped into four functional systems. Some organs work in several systems, performing different functions at different times.

- *Nutrition* (digestion): Stomach, intestines, bowel—"gut."

- *Protection*: Immune system, lymphatic fluid, bone marrow, thymus, lymph nodes, spleen; also skin, bones, muscles.

- *Communication*: "Neuro" (brain and nerves) plus "endocrine" (hormone-producing glands).

- *Detoxification* ("detox"): Mainly kidneys, liver, bladder; also skin, lungs, gut, lymphatic fluid.

We can think of ourselves as a *web* of interlinked systems. The structures (organs) of our bodies are like the strong spokes of a web; their functions are like the rings—forming interconnections, creating a cohesive whole.

The *nutrition* function occupies the central "hub" position of the web of one's being. The digestive system is the supply route of all nutrients to the entire body. Every other system is utterly dependent on it. It is generally agreed among health professionals that this system is the key to health and vitality.

The two main jobs of the digestive system are to ensure that the body is

SYSTEMS OVERVIEW

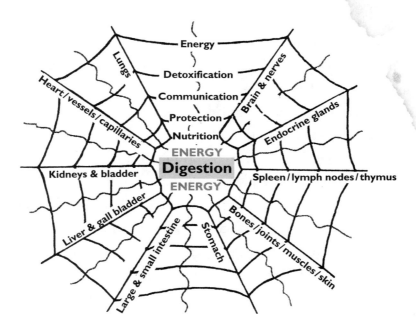

well nourished and that waste products are eliminated. It does this by producing acid and enzymes to break down foods. When healthy, it also maintains colonies of friendly bacteria that assist in protection, absorption, and "housekeeping." The benefits of a healthy digestive system are evident in adequate energy levels, good healing ability, resistance to infection, good appetite, and a healthy bowel with proper elimination of wastes. When the gut is not working well, or is overrun by unfriendly bacteria or parasites, the first signs will be a coated tongue and a general dullness in skin, hair, or eyes. If worms or other parasites are present, the child will usually have an itchy bottom and pick at nose, skin, or ears. The child may be listless and irritable, or hyperactive.

The gut has some pretty impressive workings. Enzymes are thought to be important communicators and regulators, in addition to their primary function in the process of digestion.[1] One of the stomach's main jobs is to make acid, which is used to break down foods into nutrients that are usable building blocks for repair, manufacture, growth, and protection. Foreign matter—microbes, toxins, even parasites (like worms), and bacteria—is neutralised in the stomach, provided acid production is working correctly, and has something to work on.

CHAPTER EIGHT

But our stomachs can be tricked. Things like constant gum-chewing and the continuous use of baby "pacifiers" (here in Australia they are called "dummies," maybe because they're pretty hard to talk around) give the message to the stomach to produce more acid—there is food coming!—but then all that arrives is saliva and a bit of sugar (or worse, artificial sweetener) and no solid food to attack. In the absence of food to break down, acid starts attacking the stomach lining, just as in the case of an ulcer. Next, feedback to the brain modifies acid production to preserve the lining of the stomach (also the home of "good bugs"—beneficial bacteria). The end result is a decrease in acid production, which over time can lead to an increase in microbes, and partially digested food.[2] This pattern, if repeated over time, can be the start of a serious problem.

The immune system is the central feature of the body's mechanisms for *protection*. With very close links to the gut and lungs, it is often affected by what is ingested or inhaled. As we've seen, acid in the stomach is the first line of defence against invading organisms. In addition, protective bacteria resident in the gut attack foreign invaders, and help send rejected material from food into the detox system. Approximately 70% of the immune system is found around the abdomen.[3]

The immune response involves production of specialized blood cells that, like miniature soldiers or security guards, can identify, then attack, damage, and eliminate invaders. The type of cell produced depends on the type of invader present. If overstimulated, the immune system can be a source of "friendly fire": that is, immune cells can sometimes mistakenly target and attack the body's own tissues. This overreaction is what happens in auto-immune conditions.

SYSTEMS OVERVIEW

The nervous system is involved in internal and external *communication*. Nerves bring messages to the brain and other organs, and relay commands to the muscles and other physical systems. The nervous system is particularly vulnerable to damage from nutrient deficiencies and toxins (both those generated internally and those from external sources).

The other half of the communication function is carried out by the endocrine system. Endocrine glands are specialized organs that secrete chemicals called hormones. These chemicals help coordinate and regulate many bodily functions. Hormones are involved in reproduction, growth, perception, sensory input, and metabolism. They are very potent. When no longer needed, they must be detoxed and eliminated: otherwise they can become highly toxic and wreak havoc, especially in the nervous system. Some of the most potentially dangerous toxins are derived from hormones such as cortisol and adrenalin, which are secreted during times of stress.

If the digestive system is the most important to the body, it is closely followed by the *detoxification* system. Detox involves all the various processes of neutralising and removing potentially harmful substances. Anything that enters or is produced by the body but is no longer needed must be safely eliminated by the detox system. This system includes the liver, kidneys, bladder, lungs, lymph, skin, and digestive organs. Toxins that are not neutralised and eliminated by this system become concentrated and can be very damaging.

Sources of toxins include substances added to food and drinks (intentionally or otherwise), medicines, chemicals (in foods as preservatives, additives, colourings, and agricultural residues or sprays), spent cells and hormones, and dead bacteria and other microbes, as well as their byproducts and the debris they leave when destroyed. The detox system was designed to deal with biological (occurring naturally in the outside world) and physiological

CHAPTER EIGHT

(internally produced) waste products; it is largely ineffective against synthetic, man-made products.

Stress can have a big effect on detox capability. If the daily workload is too much, the detox system will be overloaded and become less effective, allowing toxic substances to circulate and cause damage. Consider the person who, after working long hours for too many months, at first makes mistakes or sustains small injuries on the job, then falls ill and eventually burns out. Or imagine a car that is run year after year with no oil change, no tune up, no maintenance. Performance will certainly diminish; eventually the car will break down in some way.

A very important requirement for the detox system to work effectively is water. Remember, our body is made up of 80% water. Drinking two litres (quarts) of water each day is the adult requirement; proportionately less for a child.[4] By the time a person is thirsty they are usually 5% dehydrated. Very often thirst is interpreted as hunger, which can lead to overeating, thereby only adding to the dehydration. Being in a dehydrated state can affect concentration and energy levels, as toxins build up. Poor concentration and low energy can lead to further dehydration as self-care is neglected, creating a vicious cycle that results in increasing toxin levels.

Synthetic chemicals enter the food chain, and therefore our bodies, as contaminants and pollutants.

- Antibiotics (used in animals bred for meat)
- Synthetic hormones (growth stimulants used in animals)
- Herbicides (veggies, grains; sprayed onto crops)
- Pesticides
- Synthetic fertilisers
- Drugs used in animals (for worming or preventing disease in crowded conditions, and for treatment)
- Metals

SYSTEMS OVERVIEW

It is apparent that the quantity and type of pollutants in our environment has changed dramatically in the last 100 years or so. Where previously a plume of orange smoke could be seen and avoided, most of the chemicals and hazards we encounter these days are invisible and, to a large extent, undetectable. You can step around a steaming pile of horse manure, but you can't usually know whether the glass of apparently clean water you just drank was actually laced with toxic chemicals. The solution to this problem must include more than one approach. Less pollution, more good food, purer water, and healthier children are possible goals if people matter. We will focus on how to achieve the "healthier children" aspect of the solution.

ʕ ʕ ʕ

Just imagine for a moment that you are walking down the street. In one split second, you see a toddler jerk her hand out of her mother's and dash off the kerb right into the path of an oncoming bus.

Is your response distinctly separated into three reactions: one mental, one physical, and one emotional? Do you have a bit of a think about what the correct response should be? *Of course not.* Your response is all-at-once and instantaneous. Muscles are mobilised by the hormone adrenalin, which your neuro-endocrine system supplied as soon as you observed what was happening. You experience an adrenalin "rush" that gives you speed and strength for the necessary action. Your concentration is riveted on the tiny body and looming bus. Before a thought or word is formed, you race into the road and snatch the toddler out of harm's way, back to her mother's arms. She wriggles and squirms, unaware of pounding hearts, sweaty palms, and the grave danger she just escaped.

> **The beauty of human beings lies in the integration of our systems—in the harmony of everything working together.**

CHAPTER EIGHT

Separating an individual into bits to put under the microscope was the science of the last century. In this age of super-knowledge, we are beginning to realise that it's time to put it all back together, to respect the interwoven intricacies and delicate balances of the body's workings that are still a mystery.

Our systems function as one beautifully integrated whole. They are interconnected, in constant communication. It is impossible to use one part of one's self without affecting all the other parts.

- Sad news brings tears without a deliberate order.
- Food that looks appealing can bring a rumble from an empty stomach.
- A crying baby can cause milk letdown in a nursing mum—even if it's not her own baby that's crying.

Putting the individual back together gives us the advantage of acknowledging our complexity—the subjective aspects of ourselves.

Individuals are unique.

To truly represent the interconnectedness of our systems, they should be written like this:

The *nutrition-immune-neuro-endocrine-detox* system.
(And that's only some of them!)

However, we will take a look at each of these areas individually, and in more depth, in the next four chapters.

9

Nutrition

*G*rowth is the main task of childhood. During early infancy, the processes of growth and tissue repair use up 30% of the baby's total energy intake, compared to only 5% in an adult. The maximum rate of increase in brain cell numbers occurs during the first 12 months: brain cell numbers continue to increase until age two.[1] All this growth cannot happen without *food*.

Discussing the process of caring for and feeding a new baby involves some different terms. In the interest of clarity a few definitions follow:

- *Food*: Anything that animals or people eat or drink that makes them live and grow.

- *Nutrition*: The process by which living things take in food and use it.

- *Nurture*: To rear, bring up, care for, foster, or train; to nourish or feed.

- *Nourish*: To make grow or keep alive and well with food; to encourage, support, maintain, or foster.

These processes may be physical, emotional, or both. Most people would agree that love, care, and food are all pretty important for health and happiness. Just look at a baby resting on his mother's breast after a feed with a little trickle of milk slipping through the tiniest curve of a smile. Or watch a family slowing

CHAPTER NINE

down towards the end of a Christmas dinner together, savouring the contented quietness after the food is mostly gone. Is it the food, or the love, or both?

Nurturing a baby begins long before birth, through the diet of the mother. The individual mother provides the best insurance for a healthy baby by eating good food appropriate for her. The mother's nutrition during pregnancy must do the work of repair, growth, and maintenance for her own system *and* for that of her developing baby. An adequate supply of nutrients will result in strong healthy bodies for mother and child. Care in choosing whole instead of processed or packaged foods will reflect in the health of mother and baby. Even so, it is good practice for the mother to take a specially formulated vitamin and mineral supplement during preconception, pregnancy, and breast-feeding, since a slight oversupply of most nutrients will do no harm, while the deficiency of some can result in severe problems.

Having said that, we should rest assured knowing that Mother Nature amazingly provides for the survival of mothers and babies even during the most difficult situations. Although all of the scientific details may not be completely understood, it is very clear that the best choice for maintaining the health of well babies is breast-feeding, even though sometimes, when optimal nutrition for Mum is not possible, this might seem a bit like spinning straw into gold. There is no need to be concerned about producing good quality milk. With very few exceptions (which would be emphasized, if pertinent, by your health care provider), when breast milk is available it is the best choice to make.

Babies spend roughly 80% of waking time staring at their mother's face in the early stages of life. She is the new safe place: studying her face and hearing the familiar beat of her heart and the sound of her voice connect the former inner world to this challenging new outer world. From this point on, two of the most important influences in the child's life will be nutrition and nurture (through feelings of love, support, and safety). Isn't it wonderful that nature has provided both through breast-feeding?

STRUCTURE

The proper functioning of the digestive system is central for the maintenance of good health. It can be thought of as the main route through the body—a highway that brings essential nutrition in and takes waste away. It is the supply line for the entire body. By making nutrients available to organs and cells, its integrity will be reflected in the general health of the person.

As one lecturer pointed out,[2] we are all hollow in the middle like a doughnut. This design is pretty basic to most living creatures. In fact, the simplest life forms—like earthworms—are basically fancy digestive tubes.

FUNCTION

The structure of the digestive system maximizes its function every step of the way. When food enters the mouth, acid and enzymes in saliva begin to break it down into its component nutrients. The stomach continues this process of digestion, while the small intestine is involved with absorption of the nutrients into the bloodstream. The large intestine moves the unused waste products of food out of the body. The entire system is simple yet complex. Structure and function complement each other to achieve efficiency.

The digestive system relies on saliva, enzymes, acids, and *beneficial resident bacteria* to break down food, and also to defend against any harmful invaders that may enter the body through the mouth or nose. Breast-feeding supplies these beneficial bacteria, called "probiotics," if they are present in the mother. Some are found in yoghurt; some can be purchased as a powder at the health food store or chemist (pharmacy). The good ones will always require refrigeration. In bottle-fed babies, they should be introduced as a food supplement specially formulated for them.[3] These are good "bugs" that do many useful jobs, like helping the immune system keep harmful microbes and disease-causing organisms under control.

Babies are normally introduced to friendly bacteria during passage through the birth canal, when these tiny microbes enter the digestive system

CHAPTER NINE

through the mouth and attempt to set up attachment sites before the baby is exposed to unfriendly bacteria in the big outside world. Breast-feeding by a healthy mother should increase the baby's good/bad bacteria ratio, eventually establishing a colony of 99% *bifidobacterium* species in the large intestine.[4] Babies delivered by Caesarean section have not received these bacteria naturally, so should be given probiotics as a supplement from birth onwards until they maintain a colony of their own (this would be evidenced by healthy passing of stool and gastric comfort after eating).

These beneficial bacteria protect health in a variety of important ways. "Probiotic" means "life supporting," as opposed to "antibiotic," which means "able to destroy, or interfere with the development of, living organisms."

We'll digress here a little bit to ask, "What about antibiotic drugs?"

> **Using antibiotics in a severe bacterial infection is a sensible thing to do because it is frequently life-saving!**

That said, however, it must be pointed out that antibiotics are over-prescribed to a very great extent. They are often given in viral illnesses as a precaution against the *possibility* that a bacterial infection may develop in the same area affected by the virus. However, *antibiotic drugs are absolutely ineffective against viral infections.* In addition, the vast majority of viral infections in healthy individuals run their course and resolve without intervention.

The misuse or overuse of antibiotics can lead to an unhealthy intestine, because the beneficial bacteria living there are killed. Many of these drugs have side effects, including nausea, vomiting, diarrhoea, and allergic reactions, that can be very serious, especially in an infant. Use of one type by children under the age of eight can result in permanent discolouration of the teeth.[5] Other side effects include kidney and inner ear toxicity.[6]

Medical scientists have found that infants in underdeveloped countries have less allergic disease than do children in developed countries. This difference correlates to the far greater use of antibiotics in industrialised societies.[7] The World Health Organisation strongly recommends *not* using antibiotics *except for serious bacterial infections*, when, again, their use often means the difference between life and death.[8]

༺ ༺ ༺

If the "gut" does its job, neutralising harmful invaders, and fully digesting and utilising foods and nutrients, the liver has an easy time of doing *its* job, which is getting rid of unusable or harmful substances—*toxins*. Again, in addition to toxins ingested with food, these can include "biological" toxins:

- Spent hormones
- Dead, replaced cells
- Dead microbes

However, our "disposal" system stops working well and fails to keep up:

- If foods are incompletely digested.
- If internal bacteria are proliferating inappropriately [in conditions of low stomach acid found with constant "dummy" (pacifier) use, for example].
- If antibiotics wipe out protective bacteria.

༺ ༺ ༺

Digestion supports every other bodily function. To fully appreciate what is involved, we need to take a closer look at the many ways food is seen, and the many needs it can meet. Some roles food plays are physical, some emotional, and some symbolic (or spiritual).

CHAPTER NINE

In many cultures food has been regarded as a symbol of life itself ("the Bread of Life"), and as such may acquire many levels of meaning, evoking powerful emotional overtones. Indeed, the degree to which a society cares for its helpless and feeds its hungry may define its level of civilisation.

We will consider four different aspects of food:

- The nutritional value of food (quality and quantity).

- The emotional content of food ("nothing says lovin' like something from the oven").

- Food as medicine (creating health).

- Food as "the enemy" (addictions, allergy, "death by chocolate").

The first is a topic for this book; we will discuss the other three in the next book of the series, *What's Wrong with Me?*

THE NUTRITIONAL VALUE OF FOOD

The quality of the food we eat depends on the way it is grown, harvested, stored, shipped, and processed. Over the last 50 years there has been a huge decline in the nutritional value of the foods available in the marketplace.[9] The trend in western societies has been to shift away from small family farming toward enormous corporate farms and the use of sophisticated food technologies.

If the nutrients required for health are not in the foods we eat, we soon go into a deficit situation. In other words, once the savings account funds are used, all further spending goes on the credit card, which puts you deeper into debt.

Another critical factor in nutrition is how well nutrients in food are absorbed and used in your body. If they are not "bioavailable," they just taste good and pass right on through as very expensive sewage.

Third, to answer your unspoken question: No, a bottle of vitamins and minerals does not make up for a nutrient-empty diet, no matter what the advertising says. Foods need to provide macronutrients (proteins, carbohydrates, fats and oils, and fibre) and micronutrients (vitamins, minerals, trace elements, and those nutrients we haven't yet discovered or named).

More important even than food is a daily intake of water. Just water, the cleanest you can get.

These, then, are the necessary ingredients to keep a body healthy and trouble free. We require a good supply for repair, energy, growth, and protection from disease.

Every body has its particular individual needs. The more unprocessed (whole) a food is, the more likely it is that the balance and supply of nutrients will be "just right." In order to keep the body in good repair, to support growth and health at every age, we need to eat, digest, and utilise foods that are nutrient rich and suited to our individual needs. The basic types of nutrients needed are:

- Proteins, mainly for building tissue and the manufacture of hormones.

- Carbohydrates, for energy and brain function.

- Fats and oils for nerve, brain, and cellular functions, and hormone manufacture.

- Fibre, which is protective against degenerative illness.[10]

Even if the best quality nutrients are supplied in perfect balance, maintenance of health still depends on the ability of the digestive system to break down, absorb, and transport these nutrients to every part of the body where they are needed. And, like in a web, the efficiency of this system is dependent upon the integrity of all the other systems of the body.

CHAPTER NINE

PRACTICAL HELP WITH FOOD CHOICE

In addition to quality of food, the next most discussed topic would have to be quantity. How much food is enough? The answer to this age-old question lies in your hands.

Make two fists with your hands—thumbs on top. The volume of your two fists placed together approximates the volume of your stomach. Not very big, is it? This little yardstick is especially relevant for your child. Look at those two little fists and dish up a meal accordingly. Your stomach should never be stretched to hold more than that volume at any one meal, no matter how long you spent in the kitchen preparing it.

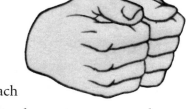

Some "bytes" (of information) about food follow:

- Drinking before, during, and after a meal contributes to overfilling of the stomach, diluting the stomach acid and diminishing its capacity to destroy harmful microbes that may be in the food.

- *Atmosphere*: Food and stress do not mix.

- *Sitting quietly*: Feeling peaceful and calm are conducive to happy, healthy mealtimes. Helping with food preparation can be a very important part of the "getting ready to eat" process, both physiologically and emotionally.

- No-one (to my knowledge) ever died from missing a meal or two. If a child isn't hungry and just plays with food, encourage another activity: rest for tiredness, exercise for relieving the "fidgets."

- Often when people feel hungry, it is a general "I want something" feeling that we automatically shove food at, when many times we are actually thirsty. In some cases, we're bored; at other times we want comfort or soothing. Distinguishing feelings is a skill that needs to be learned. If children are offered food every time they have a want, or if the adults feeding them can't help identify and name feelings, this may never be accomplished.

Feeding a family—or even one person—can be a challenge. The feeding of babies and toddlers has become an especially difficult task in these days of processed and chemically tainted foods. Babies between the ages of 6 and 18 months have an increased need for iron, zinc, B12, and calcium, as well as high requirements for protein and energy. Sue Dengate's book *Fed Up* has some wonderful suggestions for "failsafe" foods that even allergy-prone children can thrive on.[11]

The supermarket jungle is set up to entice buyers by packaging and advertising. Food has gone from a service industry to a technological industry. Attempting to read a label on a food packet feels like hearing a chemistry lecture. There are some important tools to take shopping with you. Buy foods that are as whole as possible; that is, you can see what you are buying: apples, rice, vegetables. Generally speaking, with more processing comes less nutritional value. The more numbers and chemicals you see on the label, the more you should avoid that particular food.

ABOUT FATS AND OILS

The "fat free" fad seems to have persisted past the '80s despite overwhelming evidence that fat is a vital ingredient in the body as well as in the diet. Like most things, there are good and bad choices of fats—beneficial or damaging, too much or too little.

Some of the essential uses for fats in the body are:

- As building blocks of hormones (fats and proteins are required).

- Nerves are protected by a layer of fat.

- Each cell has a membrane protecting it like a moat; membranes are made of fat.
- Our brains need fat to protect them.
- Certain fats in our blood may protect against heart and arterial disease.

The amount and kind of fats consumed can be a problem. The fats war has been raging for many years. The good fats/oils are highly beneficial and some are essential for good health. To simplify this issue, we will discuss fats from fish and plants. Each can be a source of beneficial or harmful fat.

How do I tell the good guys from the bad guys? In the good fats category, the first choice is omega 3s from fish oils (clean fish oils: our oceans are becoming so polluted with heavy metals and plastic manufacturing by-products that it is no longer safe to eat many kinds of fish). Good health food product manufacturers are distilling and purifying fish oils. Ask for clean fish oils. Fish oils are the best source of EPA and DHA (eicosapentanoic and dehydroxenoic acids) that help the body function and repair. These are especially important for children in terms of brain development and learning. It is possible to obtain omega 3 oils from plant sources, notably olive and linseed oils, but these don't have the same scope in terms of EPA/DHA action and benefit.[12]

A daily capsule of cod liver oil or halibut liver oil (first and second preference) provides protection against infection, serves as a natural source of vitamins A and D, and assists in good bone, nerve, and brain development. It is of most benefit when given daily to a child until 12 years of age. There are water-based pleasant tasting forms available now, but be sure they are from natural (not synthetic) sources.

Of course, when choosing fish to eat, the best ones are oily fish like albacore, mackerel, cold water salmon, and sardines. If in doubt about toxicity (mercury, for example), choose a smaller fish, like sardines.

HEALTH OR THE *APPEARANCE* OF HEALTH?

Do you have a slim body because of good eating and exercise, or because of starvation and amphetamines?

Do you have a happy disposition because of emotional maturity, intelligence, and good living, or because of mood-altering drugs?

Are you active and energetic due to a good night's rest and a clear conscience, or because you took stimulant drugs?

Do we as a society accept counterfeit substitutes for the real thing—replacing real food flavour and nutrition with chemical taste-alike ester-laced picture-perfect food having little nutritional value?

We eat food every day. It can contribute to vibrant good health and energy, or it can contribute to poor development and chronic ill health.

> **We should remember that, as consumers, we can have a powerful influence by the way we choose to spend our money for food.**

10

Protection: The Immune System

A child's immune system is still developing and growing.

Children have special requirements for daily routine care. Good food, rest, exercise, and love all help develop a strong immune system. When support is lacking, and challenges (such as poor diet, stress, toxicity, infections, and vaccinations) occur, the child may develop health problems, which affect immunity, digestion, behaviour, and learning.

Illness prevention is a matter of awareness, which leads to better choices. There are many ways to improve and support children's growth. Providing a good choice of healthy foods, chances for regular exercise, and lots of time to play can offset the build-up of stress and its effects. Encouraging friendships and allowing unstructured time can bring growth in social skills. Asking a child to do some work in the home (at an age-appropriate level) helps build self-esteem and life skills, as well as a sense of belonging. Time alone with each parent each day provides the support and interest that can defuse potential problems, building a relationship of trust that pays dividends in the teenage years, when challenges can create distance between parent and child. Maintaining a healthy, relaxed attitude can be a great asset for the prevention of illness and maintenance of balance in all the systems.

It is obvious to healthcare professionals how important a good start in early feeding can be for achieving good health in the years that follow. Babies who are breast-fed are in a much better position to develop good digestive and immune function.[1] The immune system is intricately involved with allergy and infections. This system needs to grow and develop properly so that the child can successfully meet the challenges of the world around him.

Healthy, normal development of the immune system has become more difficult over the last few decades because of many factors. Some of these are:

- Widespread use of strong general antibacterial disinfectants
- Earlier and multiple vaccinations
- A decrease in the nutritional quality of foods
- Increased consumption of processed foods
- Antibiotic overuse
- Toxicity and pollution in the environment
- Chemicals added to water and food
- Less exercise; more sedentary lifestyle
- Computers, TV, cars, safety issues

Before making any decisions or choices it is a good idea to understand their consequences, and what processes can be supported to achieve better outcomes in health and immunity.

STRUCTURE

What is the immune system? The immune system is not a single organ; rather, it is distributed throughout the body, and is made up of different types of white blood cells. These various cells are found in blood, liver, lymph, tonsils, bone marrow, spleen, and adenoids. Additional numbers of white blood cells can be found in almost every tissue and organ in the body. Quite a surveillance system!

This remarkable defence system has two main types of combat troops—Th_1 and Th_2—and one type of regulator—Th_3—all specialized cells called "T helper" cells.

FUNCTION

Immunity can be defined as the body's ability to resist or eliminate potentially harmful foreign material or abnormal cells. The immune system not only protects the body, it also removes waste from cells. The immune system is designed to eliminate bacteria and other microscopic invaders, such as viruses. It can attack parasites and tumours, and even prevent cancers from growing and spreading.

The first line of immune defence against foreign invaders is through a process called *inflammation*. Inflammation causes redness, swelling, itching, fever, aches, and pains.

If you cut your finger, it bleeds, and then it swells and hurts. These signs mean the immune system has been activated. Soon the bleeding slows and the cut begins to heal; the pain eventually subsides. Inflammation is a very important and necessary reaction.

How does the immune system work? Like most processes in the body, the immune system is a balancing act. It adapts to changing situations and responds accordingly. When the threat is over, it should relax back into an even balance.

Again, there are three main players in the game. Picture a seesaw balancing:

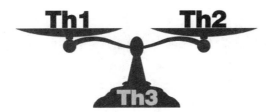

- Th1 defends against bacteria, fungi, viruses, tumours.
- Th2 defends against parasites and allergens.
- Th3 depends on correct foods.[2]

When these cells are all in balance, there is *no inflammation.* That means no redness, no swelling, no pain, no itching, no drippy nose.

CHAPTER TEN

WHAT DOES A HEALTHY IMMUNE SYSTEM NEED?

The most important aspects of daily routine for a well-tuned immune system in children include adequate sleep, clean air and water, a good healthy diet based on fresh whole foods, appropriate stress and support, healthy digestion and beneficial bacteria, exercise, and good "detox." It is very much a matter of common sense and good habits.

A breast-fed baby has immune protection in two ways. First, breast milk contains antibodies, which are nature's specifically tailored molecules created in response to a need to fight off a particular invader. So a breast-fed baby has protection from most illnesses encountered by the mother. In addition, a breast-fed baby has a stronger Th_2 position, providing the edge to start fighting any particular parasites and allergens that may be present in the environment.[3]

Enhancing this early immune-acquisition process is an extremely important part of building health in your child. There are traditional skills in nursing a child through an illness that should be known and practiced in the home and community. These require hands-on efforts involving personal choice and responsibility. Somehow our culture has been seduced into believing that drugs that suppress the symptoms of illness actually create health. Nothing could be further from the truth.

> **Every time we block the immune system (using a drug) in its effort to develop a response (like inflammation) to a particular challenge, we compromise its effectiveness.**

Obviously, in a life-threatening situation—a medical emergency—this kind of drug regimen is sometimes *absolutely necessary* for the preservation of life. But when parents who have always "soldiered on," no matter what, are required to care for a fragile new tiny person with a cold or other minor illness, they often look for the kind of solution which would allow the child to attend school or day-care instead of spending a day or two at home in bed with chicken soup, some vitamin C, and herbs for kids.

> **Suppressing symptoms is never a cure.**

The immune system takes eight days to fully respond to a challenge, with or without antibiotics or other medication. Proper care and time to recover are the only sensible options for a healthy population. Children are any nation's greatest resource.

The process of immune function, like all the other processes in the body, is highly complex, but the underlying principle is simple. Just think of the physical struggle and skills a not-yet-crawling baby demonstrates. That same process is happening in all the systems. Giving the body systems a chance to work and learn enables activation, growth, and development. These processes are the means by which children lay down the foundation for lifelong health in the first five years. A child's strength and success in these areas will define the upper limits of health and learning for the rest of life.

> **The underlying principle in health is:**
> **"Use it or lose it."**

Allowing natural processes to take their course, and supporting development, is the preferred option, interfering only when necessary, and then with caution. Growing a healthy immune system is only achieved through firsthand experience with invaders. The process of exposure to infection and overcoming it by creating antibodies leads to acquired immunity. This provides long-term (often lifelong) protection, in most cases, by expanding one's immune repertoire—enhancing the capacity of one's natural immune protection.

For this reason, be prepared to nurse your young child through a few sicknesses a year. Most people's immune systems are up and running by age 10 or 11.

CHAPTER TEN

Healthy old people generally have very strong immune systems. They will often be the only ones in the family to avoid a common cold making the rounds. This is because they already have the antibodies—the codes or formulae—to fight off that "bug," having had a similar infection earlier in life.

There are natural plants and foods that have been used as medicine for hundreds of years. These foods and herbs have proven safe and effective against most mild infections, and do not have the side effects of modern drugs. They do not interfere with the body's own defence system, so that after an illness your child has learned how to deal with the particular "bug" that caused that sickness. The next time this invader is encountered, your child will be better prepared to fight it off more quickly and easily.

- Immune system encounters a foreign invader.
- The body acts to fight and eliminate it.
- Substance is effectively eliminated.
- The body returns to balance.[4]

If this response is suppressed (remember, it requires eight days for full operation), the proper antibody encoded for that particular invading microbe will not be produced. On re-exposure to the microbe, there will be a repeat episode of illness (possibly more severe), and a second attempt to repel the invading organisms. Sometimes other agents—viral or fungal or bacterial—can now have a clearer playing field, compounding the attack. Anti*biotics* (the drugs) do not discriminate between friendly and unfriendly bacteria. They wipe out any that are present in the body except, of course, those that have developed resistance to the drug (a consequence of societal overuse). Because microbes are living organisms, they too have the ability to adapt to their environment, and do so in a matter of hours. Antibiotic-resistant strains of "bugs" are here to stay, and have become an increasingly worrisome presence.

PROTECTION: THE IMMUNE SYSTEM

The law of natural adaptation applies to all living things, including children. Prepare the child for the challenge; don't put the child in a sterile environment to prevent exposure or accident, to protect the child from being hurt. By doing so, you would also restrict healthy development.

۞ ۞ ۞

As we've said before, 70% of the immune system is located in the abdomen, near the digestive tract. The digestive and immune systems are very closely linked. The stomach is the place most foreign matter ends up (bacteria, chemicals in food). The immune system's job is to search and destroy—so why not camp on the doorstep? The immune system, like all other body systems, has specific nutrient requirements for manufacturing the defensive army of white cells. A good diet rich in fresh foods, beneficial oils, and protein is essential for immune health.

An important part of developing a strong immune system is establishing the colony of "friendly" bacteria in the digestive tract. These good bacteria are essential for the health of the entire body, playing an important part in defending and eliminating foreign invaders. New research shows that babies and children with healthy gut "bugs" have fewer infections and allergies.[5] The "good bugs" set up camp and leave no room for the "bad guys" to move in and start trouble. They produce biologically active substances that help to increase white blood cell populations. They stimulate anti-tumour activity of the specialized cell called the "macrophage," which also provides the main defence against soot, dust, and foreign particles in the lungs; these cells can simply surround and digest the offending substance! Beneficial bacteria also help correct constipation or diarrhoea by regulating the gut, provide food for other beneficial gut flora, act as a natural antacid, and help strengthen the intestinal wall.[6]

The following foods are immune boosters:[7]

- Yoghurt with potent live bacteria
- Garlic (children's formulation only)
- Raw and steamed vegetables

On the other hand, eating refined carbohydrates, found in cakes, cookies, and white bread, *depresses* the immune system within one hour.[8]

HOW DO I KEEP THE BALANCE?

For the first two years of life a baby's immune system is very much dependent on the mother providing necessary protection (antibodies) through her breast milk. Newborns exposed to a highly sterilised environment at birth lack the proper balance of "bugs" for the prevention of disease and allergies.[9] The overuse or misuse of antibiotics for infants can also lead to an unhealthy balance in the digestive tract.

The best guideline for enhancing immune function is good nutrition, adequate sleep and exercise, minimization of exposure to pollution, and appropriate interaction with the real world of people and animals and microbes. One research study showed that children living on a farm, where they had contact with dogs and pigs, had the healthiest immune systems, experiencing the fewest allergies and illnesses.[10]

A consistent finding when children are ill is that they have an immune imbalance. This imbalance is most often due to problems with the digestive system (most commonly "gut bugs" of the bad sort in the digestive tract), stress and/or toxicity, insufficient nutrients, prematurity, or low birth weight. This imbalance can lead to further reductions in gut and liver function, resulting in digestive problems, colic, diarrhoea, constipation, or reflux.

THE HYGIENE HYPOTHESIS

To develop properly, the immune system requires a clean *but not sterile* environment. Children need exposure to the real world (bugs, animals, earth, plants); temperature changes and fresh air, but not drafts or extreme weather; opportunities for the system to adapt to a variety of situations and appropriate challenges—within limits.

If provided with these conditions, a child's immune system develops resilience, adaptability, and effective responses to viral, bacterial, and environmental challenges. That is to say, the system develops "immune intelligence." If the immune system doesn't encounter the natural world, with all its microorganisms, it is stunted. Nature has created perfect timing for each skill, or capability, to develop just prior to when it's needed.

This is a good illustration of the principle of "too much, too little, just right." An old saying comes to mind: "Clean enough to be healthy and dirty enough to be happy." This is a good description of a suitable environment for happy, healthy children. In fact, with acceptance of the "hygiene hypothesis" we may need to rephrase that saying: "Dirty enough to be healthy and clean enough to find things."

The hygiene hypothesis states that in order to work, the immune system, like any other, must be challenged. In essence, that means exposure to germs and dirt, bugs and animals. Accomplishing this is something that will probably disturb most "house-proud" homemakers, but in the interest of your child's health, *let the germ-chasing go.* Exposure to environmental "bugs" and germs is the only way to build a strong immune system in a child![11]

> **Maintaining a balanced environment within our bodies is much more important for the prevention of illness than is trying to keep our air and living spaces germ-free.**

CHAPTER TEN

ALLERGY

A baby's immune system is immature at birth. The first six months appears to be a critical time; changes in the immune system occurring at that time can ultimately lead to the development of allergies.[12]

Genetic factors may be involved: if one or both parents have allergies, children are more likely to develop them as well, and they are often more severe. Factors such as presence of household smoke, either more or less than the usual number of infections, poor quality of the infant's diet, and low birth weight all seem to be related to the development of allergies.[13]

CASE STUDY

Allie and Ellie, four-year-old twin girls, became sick with stomach pains after swimming in a public pool. They were both hospitalised with massive infections in the gut. While both were very ill, Ellie reached the point of being in danger of losing her life. They both survived, but when I first saw them, they had never completely gotten over the physical and emotional consequences of the incident.

There were many children in the pool that day, all swimming in the same contaminated water. Why didn't the others get ill after exposure to the same bugs? The answer, of course, lies in the protective mechanisms of their digestive and immune functions.

In the healthier children, the gut barrier (mucosa) would have been stronger and contained adequate numbers of protective bacteria. The stomach acid may have been more effective. Colonies of protective bacteria would have triggered immune responses to deal with the invaders. In other words, their systems carried out their functions, performing as they should.

Following treatment, the girls now have healthy, fully functioning immune and digestive systems. They are no longer troubled by off-and-on symptoms of gastric distress, allergic reactions, or recurrent infections.

11

Communication: The Neuroendocrine System

(In plain English: Nerves and hormones)

Nerves and hormones have many jobs. In addition to allowing us to communicate with each other, one of their most important functions is *internal* communication. Nerve impulses and chemical communicators are the vehicles the body uses to regulate its workings. Nerves enable us to observe and learn about the world outside. They carry information—from sensors in the eyes, ears, skin, nose, and mouth—to the brain, which then interprets these messages as sight, sound, touch, smell, and taste. After this selective perception, the brain may stimulate the production of hormones. These hormones might be beneficial "feel good" hormones, like endorphins, or anxiety-provoking, like adrenalin, stimulating fear and flight responses. The "neuro" and "endocrine" systems are so intimately linked that it would be hard to study one without also examining the other.

STRUCTURE

What is the neuroendocrine system? "Neuro" refers to nerves, which align themselves in a network that links all parts of the body to the brain using energy—electrical, chemical, and, perhaps, other forms of energy. They communicate with each other by releasing small "neurotransmitter" molecules directly into the tiny spaces between nerve cells.

"Endocrine" refers to chemical messengers produced in specialized glands or nerve cells that travel through the body in the blood, regulating and coordinating various functions at points distant from where they are made. These include hormones and possibly other chemical messengers.

The nervous system can be compared to a communication system that includes a variety of ways to deliver messages throughout a building. There are similarities to telephones, fibreoptic cables, computers, and televisions, and to the different kinds of relay networks linking every part of the system.

Nerve fibres are coated with a fatty protective covering, called a "myelin sheath." The coating is made from, and kept in good repair by, the good oils (that is, omega 3 oils, particularly from fish) we consume.

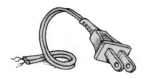

Bundles of nerve fibres inside the protective covering are very sensitive to damage from any toxins present in the body.

FUNCTION

Nerves are responsible for voluntary and involuntary events.

- *Voluntary*: Movement (muscles are stimulated).

- *Involuntary*: Breathing, heart beating, digesting food, liver and kidneys cleansing the blood.

Even while asleep, essential functions operate without conscious effort.

The neuroendocrine system is probably the most complex of all the systems. It provides the mechanism by which we *feel* and *perceive*. It is invisible, and is perhaps the most vulnerable of all the systems, yet is arguably the one having the greatest impact.

Hormones regulate communication; good news travels as fast as bad news.

COMMUNICATION: THE NEUROENDOCRINE SYSTEM

Hormones create the wide variety of emotions—everything from ecstasy to despair, and all feelings in between.

When observing new surroundings with friends, have you ever wondered why you noticed the paintings on the wall, while someone else noticed the plants or the photos?

Our nervous systems cannot take in everything at once; rather, we scan the outer world selectively based on wiring hook-ups, internal patterns, and past experience. Hormones unite the body, working with the nerves to form a cohesive network that allows us to react as an integrated entity.

> **The neuroendocrine system interlinks and influences all systems.**

Each cell of our body can receive and read messages through its highly selective set of "receptor" molecules. *They are highly selective:* there is far too much information to receive it all. In this way we choose what to focus on, and can reinforce those choices.

Many neurotransmitters are very small molecules called peptides. In the book *Molecules of Emotion*, Candace Pert explains that these peptides select which information will be received and processed, and which will be ignored. If you have ever been upset and in a hurry and wasted a half-hour looking for keys to the car that were right under your nose, you will understand the term "domestic blindness" and the concept of "selective neuropeptides," because you have experienced both firsthand.

In a word jumble, if you are looking for a particular word (say, "fun"), your whole system will be tuned in and scanning for "fun."

You will perceive other words as your eyes scan and

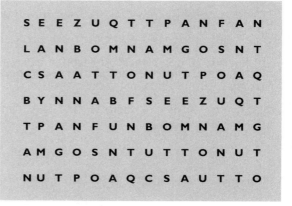

match, but the aha! comes when you see the word "fun." This same process is used as we think about certain things over and over again. We selectively "program" (or make it easier to see) what we expect to see. This principle plays an important role in bonding, recognition, and learning. If I expect to find a task easy, it usually is; if I expect to find it impossible, then that is usually the case.

The good part about this process is that we can actually influence the way we see the world; and it's never too late to change our minds in terms of attitude (or what we expect to see).

Some scientists say hormones *are* emotions. Again, in *Molecules of Emotion,* Candace Pert speaks of learning emotions and taking responsibility for how we feel and act.[1] We can *choose* how we feel. It takes practice and determination, but it is definitely possible.

Daniel Goleman, in *Emotional Intelligence,* makes the point that our emotional skills and integrity are some of the best indicators for success in life's ventures. The most influential time for learning values by "modelling" is before the age of six. Modelling refers to the learning of behaviours through exposure, imitation, and, ultimately, ownership and internalization. Emotional states are learned by *feeling* them, not by understanding through verbal descriptions.[2]

WHAT DOES THE HEALTHY NEUROENDOCRINE SYSTEM NEED?

The good fats—olive oil, fish oils, monounsaturated oils—are essential for nerve function, and play a protective role. They are also essential for the manufacture of hormones. Hormones are made out of protein and fat. "Bad fats" (animal fats, palm oil, cottonseed oil) can become free radicals when heated, or by conversion in the body. These damage otherwise healthy cells, including nerves.

Nerves are extremely vulnerable to the effects of toxins. If stress hormones are not eliminated, after a time they become capable of doing damage to the nerves in ways that can be as harmful as damage caused by chemicals from outside the body.[3] This is especially true when the stress goes on for a long period of time, or is intense or traumatic. A build-up of stress hormones adds to the load of the detox system. When the detox system is overloaded, toxins can recirculate; these are now more powerful and more damaging, as if they had been concentrated.

When this happens, the result can be inflammation. Sometimes this immune response becomes overactive, causing all sorts of problems, like eczema, asthma, and allergy. Damage to nerves could lead to conditions such as hyperactivity, learning problems, ADD, and autism. The accuracy and health of the connections between nerves and brain can diminish in function, resulting in blocks, distortions, and even reversals of learning and information storage.

Once we begin discussing stress and hormones we've stepped out of the structural realm and into the thin air of the *functional* arena: the unseen and largely immeasurable.

The body is set up to respond to threats or danger by reacting quickly with "alerting" hormones.

A small stress should produce a small response; a large stress should evoke a large response. Once someone is exposed to too many sensitising factors, however, small stresses start to provoke exaggerated responses. The appropriate small response is replaced with an "over-the-top" large response. Subsequently, even very small irritants or annoyances can continue to provoke magnified responses.

Behaviours such as aggression, anxiety, depression, learning problems, and self-control issues can all be related to malfunctions of the nervous system. Therefore, keeping our finely tuned nervous systems healthy is critical for managing our reactions to stress within an acceptable range. Once stress or sensitising factors become "too much," the nervous system is vulnerable to damage, which can result in diminished function.

There are positive strategies for intervening in these situations that can make a huge difference, and the earlier they are employed the better. We've explored the way the immune system needs the stress of microbial attack to activate and develop properly. The nervous system too needs practice through stimulation. Babies always seem to sleep better in households with normal noise levels, tending to wake up in dead silence. They also need to learn to relax when soothed and comforted.

We have seen how internal drives and wants and needs result in the development of muscles, skills, growth, and learning.

> **Stress, within parameters healthy for the individual, is not the enemy, but rather is an essential part of life.**

Chemicals of communication contribute to our unique personalities. As we grow and develop, each of us forms our own view of the world and the people in it. Every learning process is individualized by each person's brain chemistry, which in turn is supported by all systems of the body. Experiences, opportunities, and attitudes of the child, family, and community all play a role in the finished product—which, when supported properly, will be a generation of happy, healthy, intelligent children.

12

Detoxification

The processes in the body that eliminate harmful materials—toxins—are collectively called the detoxification, or "detox," system.

WHAT IS A TOXIN?

"Toxin" is another name for a poison. A toxin is any substance that is not needed in the body. These can be very damaging.

DOES EVERYONE HAVE TOXINS?

We are all exposed to toxins every day. They can simply be material our body no longer needs. We are constantly making new cells and replacing old ones. The old ones need to be eliminated. Other sources of internally generated toxins are the stomach, and used hormones. We produce hormones all the time to enable growth, sleep, and response to stress. When these internal chemical substances have done their job, they need to be eliminated too. It's like the garbage bin filling up . . . you need to empty it regularly. Naturally produced toxins are easier for our systems to eliminate than unnaturally produced synthetic chemical toxins.

WHERE ELSE DO TOXINS COME FROM?

Toxins can also enter into the body from the environment: most take the form of chemicals added to what we eat and drink. They can also be in the air

CHAPTER TWELVE

we breathe: pollution of all kinds—cigarette smoke, pesticides, chemical cleaners, and traffic fumes. Unnatural pollutants like these are harder for our bodies to eliminate.

Getting rid of all kinds of toxins should be a natural part of our day. The liver and kidneys, the lymphatic system, even our lungs and skin all help us to detoxify potentially harmful material. But if there is *too much* toxic material, our bodies can't keep up. Then we may begin to perform less efficiently.

To illustrate, let's consider the common household steam iron. I'm sure most people have at some time ignored the instruction "distilled water only," and have instead added tap water to a steam iron. The water *looked* perfectly clear. But eventually the little holes in the iron became clogged up with flaky white bits, which are minerals from the tap water that accumulated as more and more tiny particles stuck together while the water evaporated. The result was spotty shirts (especially the dark colours where the white flecks showed up dramatically) and blobs of water spurting out where a fine mist of steam should have been. The steam iron just wasn't doing the job it used to. Performance was certainly affected—and badly. Yet the iron itself was still working well. It used the electricity—no shorts, no breaks in the wires; it heated to the right temperature and adjusted it appropriately; the parts were not loose, or falling off, or catching on the fabric. But a substance that should never have gone in gummed up the works. So we now have an iron contaminated by toxins.

WHAT TO DO ABOUT IT?

Detoxing the steam iron would involve using a steam iron cleaner, which loosens the scaly bits and flushes them out.

Our systems can become "toxic," or overloaded with toxins, just like the steam iron. The toxins can then affect any system in our body, interfering with the way it works.

Some of the short-term effects people experience can be:[1]

- Allergies
- Bowel problems (diarrhoea or constipation)
- Tiredness, sore muscles
- Stomachache, nausea, indigestion, vomiting
- Headache
- Poor memory
- PMT (premenstrual tension)

If these toxins persist long-term, they become more concentrated. They are stored in fat cells, where levels build up. When we go for a long time without eating (say overnight while asleep), some of these are released along with the fat we must use to provide us with energy. Our body now tries to detox again; but the toxins become more concentrated and exert a stronger effect with each attempt. You may wake up in the morning feeling really tired and weak, with a funny taste in your mouth and a headache.

HOW DOES THE BODY GET RID OF TOXINS?

Most toxins enter the body through our food and water. The internal systems they pass through all have ways of eliminating some of them.

- *Mouth*: Saliva is acidic, helping to kill bacteria and microbes.

- *Stomach*: Acid, enzymes, and good bacteria all help break down and eliminate toxins.

- *Immune system*: Again, 70% is around the digestive tract to help attack and eliminate toxins.

- *Liver*: Has the main job of breaking down toxins into harmless waste that is flushed out of the body.

This specialized defence system deals very effectively with toxins. It is, quite simply, amazing.

However, *the key to maintaining excellent health* is to have even fewer toxins than our body can comfortably cope with. When this is the case, we can use the major part of our nutrients for repair and functioning at peak levels.

Problems start when our toxic load becomes much greater than what our body is able to eliminate. The short- and long-term consequences start to become noticeable. Often people will say, "I just can't do as much as I used to."

Or, "I'm tired by lunch time."

Or, "I seem to catch every 'bug' that comes along."

When people have too many toxins in their body they can become "sensitive" to other chemicals in our food, water, and/or environment.

CASE STUDY: COREY, AGE 6

Corey developed problems with his skin (eczema) and food sensitivities when he was a baby. His ability to tolerate certain foods was limited. Each year he became more reactive to a longer list of foods and plants. With guidance in food choices and some herbal medicines his system came into a more effective balance.

When Corey stopped eating lots of wheat and cheese, his eczema cleared up. After he was "desensitised," he could have these foods every once in a while, and the eczema didn't come back.

> **If a child becomes sensitive to chemicals, his nutrient stores are affected.**

However, when Corey's family relocated, he changed schools and he ate too much sugar (chocolate, lollies, fizzy drinks). The eczema just wouldn't go away, and he began to have one "cold" after another.

When spring/summer came he developed hayfever (remember, wheat is a grass), and now, in addition to the eczema, his eyes itched and his nose dripped a lot.

Corey made an appointment and had a "tune-up." He took some herbs formulated specifically for children. His diet improved, he drank more water, and he took some homoeopathic drops, all of which helped his body detox. Within three or four weeks he was feeling much better and his symptoms were almost gone.

TOXINS AND SENSITIVITIES (REACTIONS)

Imagine that the jar represents your body's upper limit for dealing successfully with toxins. As you come into contact each day with toxins in the air (microbes, pollutants, car fumes), in the water (chemicals like fluoride and chloride, and pollutants), and in food (sprays, chemicals, additives, and colourings), drop by drop the jar gets full . . .

The body can only handle so much in a day. When the jar is filled right up to the top, what happens when the next drop is added? It spills over and you may have a "reaction"—a symptom telling you that something is wrong. The most common ones are tummy aches, asthma, headaches, learning and memory problems, poor concentration, skin rashes, tiredness, and irritability.

Some chemicals have very powerful effects on nerves and hormones, and can cause reactions such as aggression, hostility, mood swings, depression or teariness, anxiety, and fearfulness.

This is because the nerves are easily affected by toxins. In fact, while toxins have a variety of negative effects on many parts of the body, it is often the nervous system that exhibits signs first.

All toxins are neurotoxic (cause damage to nerve cells).[2]

CHAPTER TWELVE

WHAT CAN I DO TO HELP MY BODY STAY TOXIN-FREE AND HEALTHY?

There are lots of things we can do to help our bodies stay healthy. One of the best ways is to *avoid* toxins whenever you can.

Don't:

- Don't stay around cigarette smoke and car fumes (especially in an enclosed space like a shed or garage).

- If you're using chemicals (household cleaning products, bleach, fly killer, weed killer, spray paints, or oil-based paints) make sure you don't touch the chemicals, inhale the fumes, or get any of it on your skin.

- Some plastic drink bottles are not meant to be reused. When they are washed in hot soapy water they may release toxic fumes and chemicals into the next drink you put in that bottle. To be safe, always use plastic intended for food and that is identified as suitable for reuse.

- *Putting anything on your skin is the same as eating it—make sure it's not poisonous!* Any product applied to the skin—makeup, shampoo and conditioners, perfume, soaps, and oils—all need to be scrutinized. *Mineral oils, even some baby oils, are petroleum-based products. Lotions and creams made from vegetable oils are preferred for skin care of babies and small children.*

Do :

- Eat unprocessed foods as much as you can. These are the foods that don't need a packaging label, because they haven't been changed by processing—foods like fruit, vegetables, rice, nuts, and beans. Wash produce in clean water before eating, just in case it has been sprayed.

DETOXIFICATION

- Drink lots of water—just water.

- Avoid caffeine (including cola drinks).

- Avoid artificial sweeteners, which may have subtle effects in developing brains and in brains of long-term users. These were approved for use in spite of evidence that they are linked to the development of brain tumours in laboratory rats.[3]

- Avoid refined sugar and sweet things like cakes, cookies, ice cream.

Fruit, veggies, nuts, and whole grains all contain natural antioxidants and vitamins and minerals. If you eat plenty of these types of foods, they actually clean up and flush toxins out of your body. These foods act as a sponge to eliminate toxic waste.

Your liver is one of the most important organs in your body (maybe the most important) because one of its jobs is to clean up toxins to prevent damage. A healthy liver filters toxins out of the blood as it passes through, changing them into forms that are safe to eliminate from your body. A sick or overtired liver won't be able to do this work, and toxins will recirculate with uncleansed blood, allowing them to cause more damage as they proceed. The ability to detox can vary sixty-fold within a small group of people. Remember *individual differences*. The outcome following exposure to a toxin will depend on the particular day, time, and activity level of each person. A critically important factor in determining whether there will be a toxic overload is the amount of stress present.

It is important to keep in mind that symptoms of food, or other, sensitivity can begin *up to 72 hours after exposure* to the offending substance.

Imagine one day a person eats and sleeps well, exercises, drinks plenty of water, and has a happy, stress-free day. The ability to detox chemicals and other harmful substances encountered during this day will be in top form (excellent!). And yet, on another day, the same person could be exposed to a smaller toxic load, but because of sickness, lack of sleep, too much stress, no food or—worse—poor food choices,* will have a severe sensitivity reaction.[4]

> **It is all a matter of balance.**

The greater the ability to eliminate toxins, the greater is the probability of seeing a healthy, happy child.

---

* Generally speaking, we in the Western world suffer from "over-consumption malnutrition"—"too much" of empty calories, not "too little" of good food. It is in this context that I have made this statement, and do not intend in any way to be insensitive to the needs of those in the world who experience hunger, or even starvation, on a daily basis.

13

Stress: The Driving Force in Life

Stress is one of the most important aspects of life. It is the thread that runs through it all—from the little sperm swimming, to birth and growth and learning, to the moment of a final breath. It's the spark that drives all of our systems, our adaptations—our survival. It is a basic energy link, and it needs to be acknowledged. Stress is what drives the healing process. It is not given the credit it deserves. Drugs don't heal. A person heals because he or she has the will to live, and can meet stress and respond to it. This could be why some cases of recovery happen in the face of a "terminal" illness.

Let's get this concept out there for discussion and review in terms everyone understands. Even vegetables respond to drought and insects, and sometimes survive. Stress is a powerful tool that we have been afraid to use.

EXPERIENCING STRESS IS ESSENTIAL FOR HEALTH

According to Mosby's Medical Dictionary,[1] "stress" can be defined as any emotional, physical, social, economic, or other factor that requires us to make a response or a change. Any factor that causes stress can be named a "stressor." Interestingly, stress can arise from devastating, challenging, or *joyful* experiences; what makes an event stressful is that it requires change or adaptation. So, marriage, death of a loved one, divorce, the birth of a baby, and moving to a new home *all* fall into the "high stress" category.

One easy-to-remember guideline for assessing the level of stress is to consider an individual's ability to experience a given amount of stress over a given amount of time without developing any negative long- or short-term consequences. Each person will have their "too much," "too little," and "just right" parameters for dealing with stress.[2]

In the following case, stress was the force that drove Rachel to search out a different approach to the birth of her second child. It resulted in a happy ending, certainly with a reduction in stress to more appropriate levels for all concerned.

CASE STUDY: RACHEL AND HENRY

Rachel was a lovely but very worried mother, with a small baby and a big belly, who came looking for hope. As her story unfolded, Rachel's fear of her upcoming second delivery was explained. Her first pregnancy and Henry's birth had been one long nightmare. Henry had needed extraordinary medical intervention to survive. Mother and baby had been separated by medical procedures for months. This first birth experience left Rachel feeling helpless, depressed, and frightened. Henry had many health issues that persisted into his second year.

When I saw her, Rachel had two goals. One was to do everything possible to help Henry get well by using natural therapies; the other was to have a safe, successful second pregnancy, ending with the delivery of a healthy baby. The medical practitioners she had consulted prior to our visit had offered little hope of anything but a rerun of her bad experience with baby number one.

Happily, with dietary and lifestyle changes and herbal treatment for stress, the outcome was successful. No toxaemia or high blood pressure developed, so intervention for these was not necessary. We ended up having a healthy baby delivered, without incident, to a healthy, happy mother.

Supporting and assisting natural growth processes is the preferred and safest way of achieving health at all ages. Extraordinary and highly technical interventions can be life-saving when required; but prevention and support can, in most instances, make pregnancy and childbirth the joyful, natural process it is meant to be. The stress of having a second child in the home can then be taken in stride, because ability to adapt successfully will have been enhanced.

During the birth process, many triggers for development are set in motion. The mother and baby are in constant communication through hormones produced by each. Experiencing the stress of labour is a necessary process—essential for preparing the new baby to function independently after birth. New tasks will include breathing; body temperature control; changes in the way the heart pumps blood; adapting to light and sound at new, intense levels; and supporting the body's weight under gravity without the benefit of freely floating in a watery environment.

Again, it is amazing to note that nature has provided the perfect antidote to the stress of birth. If the baby is placed at the mother's breast immediately after birth, before expulsion of the placenta, hormones that result in relaxation and feelings of safety are triggered in both mother and newborn. The length of the umbilical cord is about 26 inches, exactly what's required for a baby to comfortably reach mother's breast. The stimulus of the infant nursing benefits the mother. Hormones are produced that signal the placenta to close off the blood supply and so prevent haemorrhage. Early suckling also stimulates the contractions necessary for delivery of the placenta. This usually takes 15 to 20 minutes. Just enough time to soothe and relax a stressed mother and baby, and to create a nursing bond. This short amount of time is crucial for both, as it becomes one of the most important events for future reference when dealing with stress encountered later in life. Both learn that once stress is over their bodies will release the "relax and feel good" hormones. For the baby, this early learning leads to the creation of trust, security, and safety in mother's arms.

After this initial process of settling and bonding (which may or may not include father and others for support), father, siblings, and grandparents can be introduced, but need to remember that all these new experiences are highly stimulating and tiring after such an arduous journey. Mainly what mother and baby need most is sleep, quiet, and a DO NOT DISTURB sign hung on the front door. It certainly isn't the time for lots of visitors or invasive procedures.

Whether or not the baby continues with breast-feeding is the next critical factor in how the management of stress is learned. The hormones released with the milk letdown response act as a relaxant, for both mother and child, and provide a healing, soothing means of repair and learning for both. Time spent breast-feeding enhances bonding between mother and child, allowing for positive communication and a safe, comforting experience.

There is another factor having to do with stress and health that should be mentioned here. During a baby's period of growth inside the womb, there is a critical time when the mother's hormones trigger a "set-point" for the baby's stress response. The baby's nervous system "assumes" that this level of hormone activation is "normal." This explains in part why some babies are so relaxed and "laid back," while other babies are highly stressed even just hours after birth.[3]

A mother who is relaxed, happy, and well cared for will have hormones that produce, on the whole, beneficial mood states. The baby experiences a "normal" state of relaxation and contentment for most of the time spent in the womb. This general relaxed state of well-being becomes the functional setting for the developing nervous system.

When mothers are anxious, fearful, stressed, and/or malnourished, the hormones produced are anxiety-provoking, bathing the baby in messages of stress, fear, and alarm. The set-point for this child will be much higher than that of a relaxed crib-mate.

> **Stress itself is an essential response. How an individual responds to stress is determined by many factors, including present state of health, inherited systems, diet, exercise, and lifestyle, to name a few.**

The appropriate stress level will, of course, vary with different circumstances and stages of development, and for each child, will be influenced by set-point. Like everything having to do with health, stress is a matter of "too much," "too little," or "just right." At birth, stress is physical; it stimulates and alerts the baby to prepare to acquire the massive new learning necessary to make the shift from dependent foetus to functioning newborn. As expected, each child will behave very differently from birth onwards. Some develop an appropriate response to stress: that is, a small stress produces a small response; while others become "hypersensitive": a small stress produces a *big* response.

It is interesting to observe how some babies learn to soothe themselves, while others get more and more wound up, and can't seem to settle without help—sometimes even *with* help. Some studies[4] have suggested that learning how to soothe and comfort the self is a skill that anxious babies don't learn: thus, the gap between the "sleep through anything" babies and the "highly strung, oversensitive" babies grows wider over those first five years.

Remember, we must always keep the issue of individual differences in mind.

CASE STUDY: NON-IDENTICAL TWIN GIRLS, NELL AND JACKIE

Nell was born first; her delivery was uneventful and brief. She received good care from her mother and the attending staff. Nothing out of the ordinary occurred during delivery or afterward. However, Jackie, her twin, became "stuck" in a horizontal position across her mother's abdomen during labour, waiting to be born. It was a tight squeeze; she was finally delivered, after an exhausting struggle, with mechanical assistance. Her mother referred to it as "dragged out." Jackie was then poked and tested and separated from mother, wired for vital signs, and, in every way imaginable, placed in highly stressful circumstances.

Their shared time *in utero* provided these girls with nearly identical environments with respect to stimulation, support, and experience. However, the first twin was stressed from before birth, while the second twin, who underwent much more painful and invasive interventions during and after delivery, was quite unaffected by all the drama.

What can we learn from our twins, Nell and Jackie? They shared the same pregnancy and the same hormones, but had different stress levels.

In this case, their physical systems (from genetic inheritances as different as those of any two siblings) made the critical difference. Nell, the first-born, was much more sensitive; she had a fragile constitution and was affected by any stress much more than Jackie. Even an ordinary, uneventful birth process was traumatic for her. Jackie, on the other hand, experienced a very difficult birth, but took it all in stride. She was stimulated, but not stressed.

> **Individual differences will determine whether an event is experienced as stress or challenge. Every child is unique.**

Remember the POD—the Personal Observation Dome? Varying experiences all become part of the child's unique way of observing the world. A developing sense of safety or apprehension will be carried as a filter into new experiences. The library of events—interactions and experiences, positive and negative—thus created is stored in nerve-brain-chemistry-cell structures. Every time a primary learning experience is taken off the shelf and remembered, it becomes more vivid, more intensely personalized, and more deeply internalized as being *true*. Patterns of behaviour evolve in response, and expectations become part of the child's "self-talk." The creation of models and players in the internal dialogue contributes to our view of the world and life in general. These are the building blocks of *attitude*.

What we choose to remember (and *that* is always selective) will develop into an outlook, or orientation, that becomes part of our personality. There are several critical times during development and growth when the element of choice affords opportunities to enhance attitude—the ability to see positives rather than negatives.

TOO MUCH STRESS IS HARMFUL

Hormones are powerful chemicals produced by our endocrine glands. When we experience extreme, prolonged stress, they can become quite toxic.

As we've seen, stress is a necessary and important part of how our bodies work. The hormones produced in response to stress give us an immediate extra burst of strength and energy, allowing us to escape danger.

In a book by Robert Sapolsky called *Why Zebras Don't Get Ulcers*,[5] the author explains that when a lion chases a herd of zebra, all the animals are pumping out stress hormones like mad, running like their lives depend on it (which, for both species, is true). But the race is quite short; as soon as the single, unlucky zebra is down, and the lion is happily enjoying lunch, all the other zebras calm down, and after a short time are grazing peacefully again. Their systems have switched to an "all's well" mode, are producing calming hormones, and they are soon back to normal.

Why is it that one person is affected and another person not affected by the same situation? One part of the answer is that stress is a matter of perception. The interpretation of an event determines whether that stress does or does not become an issue. Stress is also a biochemical event. Stress becomes a problem when there is too much, too little, or never-ending pressure. When there is no way to adapt, resolve, or repair a situation, stress and pressure are magnified. This can create feelings of helplessness, guilt, depression, victimization, or worthlessness.

Ongoing, unrelenting stress can be damaging in a "too much" sense; there are also situations when there is "too little" time for recovery.

Physical example: One night of broken sleep or too much activity can be made up over the next few days. When sleep is missed night after night, stress builds up in the form of internal chemicals (hormones and toxins) that begin to damage the systems. Signs of an increasing stress response can be irritability, impaired judgment and performance, and even overreactions (in a physical sense).

Emotional example: Everyone has worried about something, at some point in life. This type of stress can be short-term, perhaps motivating us to work harder, or it can be long-term and exhausting, preventing a good result. It all depends on the individual's perception and neurochemistry. Some people do their best work under pressure, while others freeze and draw a blank when stressed.

ANXIETY

When stress becomes a reaction to an event or concern that may (or may not) occur at some future time, it is called anxiety. It is a type of stress we humans create for ourselves; it is a characteristic that can be acquired before birth.[6] It is the kind of stress involved when someone dreads a course or a teacher, and may go on every day for a year, in and out of the classroom. Many times anxiety is created when we think back to stressful events, reliving those memories. When anxiety persists even in times of attempted relaxation, the body chemistry matches that of the stressful situation. An anxious person responds as if he or she were actually in the imagined setting or experience.

This kind of stress is ongoing and damaging, because soon the chemicals being overproduced become "too much" to eliminate and are toxic. The result may be that one physical system after another diminishes in function.

It doesn't help that the media (TV, newspapers, movies) tend to sensationalize (even exaggerate), often focusing on the most shocking and negative events from around the world, which come blasting right into your living room (car, walkman, computer). This "saturation negativity" can result in daily doses of stress, keeping the systems on full alert with no relief. One way to describe stress is: *High responsibility with no control.*

We can't really do much about wars, famines, earthquakes, and violence, but being constantly bombarded with so much information is almost like being there—and the helpless feelings generated are translated into the release of stress hormones. When present most of the time, these, and the changes in the body that happen because of them, have serious effects that can eventually affect the brain and its ability to receive information accurately.

COPING WITH TOO MUCH STRESS

There are natural ways to release the stresses that we internalize. These techniques are familiar to almost everyone. Children provide some of the best examples of stress release in action. When a child falls or is hurt in some way, the first response is to find Mother, to allow her to comfort and reassure and even kiss away the hurt. What happens in this "magic moment"? An emotional, or even physical, pain is transformed by loving actions and words into a smile. What a great definition of stress release. Pain and stress hormones are blocked by a flood of feel-good hormones generated by Mother's loving kindness.

If you have ever been frustrated or disappointed, or had an argument or conflict with a friend, you may have gone for a walk to "blow off steam" or "think it out." Working out at the gym or spending some time in a creative activity, such as pottery or woodworking, are all natural ways people release stress.

Biological studies of stress have provided evidence that it can make an enormous contribution to disease and ill health. It makes sense that the reverse would also be true: the appropriate and swift release of stress can contribute to health and well-being.[7]

"WHAT CAN I DO TO HELP ME RELAX AND NOT STRESS OUT?"

You can help yourself in many ways. Some suggestions are listed here:

- *Do physical exercise* that you enjoy. This is one of the best and easiest ways to release stress and keep it from building up.

- *Eat healthy whole foods* (*not* processed).

- *Drink plenty of plain water* with nothing added—ideally at least 1.5 to 2 litres (quarts) a day.

- *Learn to create positive thoughts* and pictures in your mind. This gets easier with practice. Choose one or two of your happiest memories, and then spend a few minutes reliving them. Your body will respond as though they were actually happening, and will start creating healthy "feel good" hormones. It's a great way to balance your energy too.

- *Stay in the present.* Most stress is about what has already happened (embarrassing moments or mistakes) or fears about the future (what's going to happen). Again, in both situations, you are really powerless *now* because you can't *do* anything to change that event. Staying in the present at least allows you to take action—to *do* something—and that in itself releases stress.

- *Choose positive feelings.* You can learn to create happy, positive feelings that build good health, or you can cop out and believe "I can't change," "I can't help the way I feel," or "I'm just a moody, negative person." *You* are in charge because of the thoughts *you* create.

The choice is yours.

14

Wiser Choices

People develop different ways of looking at life, different *attitudes* toward life.

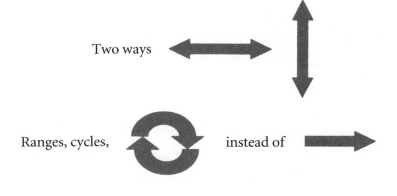

Two ways

Ranges, cycles,   instead of

Some people picture life as a one-way journey.

Some picture life as a ladder.

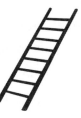

Some prefer the image of a spiral revolving in cycles.

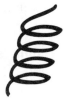

CHAPTER FOURTEEN

At some time we all fall into the trap of "if only."

- "If only I had a new car."
- "If only my boss appreciated me or paid me more money."
- "If only my children weren't so demanding or difficult."

The assumption is that then life would be better or easier, and we would be happier.

> **The expectation that everything should be perfect all the time is the surest way I know to become stressed and ill.**

Let's imagine there is no sickness in the world. What would children (and parents) need to reach their full potential? What would they need to be happy? Children would still need love and guidance and support and training. There would still be times of conflict and growth through painful experiences and wrong choices. When the burden of ill health is added, everything becomes more difficult, and problems seem magnified.

Things don't make people happy. People have the responsibility to create their own happiness. Having achieved that, circumstances—good or ill—can then be experienced as lessons to learn from, and to grow through.

We all have the ability to influence others *and ourselves* by the choices we make. This is particularly true in terms of understanding, comfort, and appreciation, which can be conveyed easily through a hug or a kind smile. These means of communication have benefits throughout the entire human system, all delivered through the nerves and hormones. A simple touch can have an actual healing, therapeutic action within the body.

Happiness and joy are usually found in relationships and in service to others. Feelings like belonging, acceptance, love, kindness, and trust are all contributors to happiness. Those feelings are experienced most often in a loving family, and are best when mutual. Children learn happiness from being with happy people, and they learn sadness from being with sad people.

Emotions drive learning.[1]

Learning is very much a mind/body experience.

Intention comes from within.

Interaction takes place outside in the world.

New experiences are then integrated and interpreted within.

Drive . . . interaction . . . integration.

> **Experience is still the best teacher.**
> **When adults learn to find joy in what they have, rather than longing for what they don't have, children will too.**

EPILOGUE

A Job Well Done

We arrived at Sydney International Airport hours before the flight would board. We wandered around looking at shops and food offerings, settling for I-don't-remember-what at a salad bar. As the minutes ticked by, conversation gradually wound down to an awkward silence.

There was no more to do or say—the last of the responsibilities for my son's life to date were neatly tucked in his carry-on.

Lost in our own thoughts, we walked to the customs hall, coming to a stop at the glass doors. I silently admired the handsome young man in the suit who stood before me. Teacher, musician, bushman, brother; a son to make any mother proud. He was now leaving for America, 10,000 miles away—ironically my homeland—with three phone calls in the two years of his mission to look forward to. Letters of course—but they aren't in the now, are they?

Hugs and "I love you" over, I stood watching his easy walk—shoulders squared, no hesitation, no backward glance.

I realised then I had done my job well. As tears blurred the departure schedule, another piece of my heart went with him.

Parenting is the only job I know of that—when done well—leaves you totally and utterly alone. He'll come back to visit as a friend, but the child has become a man in his own right, and the little boy is gone . . . forever.

Bittersweet—yes.

EPILOGUE

But the true reward lies in becoming part of the next cycle of life, which brings with it precious new babies to love, to expand your heart—grandchildren, who remind you of every sweet moment you ever had with your own children in a smile, a tear, a giggle, a hug. The missing piece is given back. Memories and love are magnified tenfold, until the joy becomes almost more than you can bear—powerful emotion that is, in fact, very reminiscent of the loss.

A life in review contains the fullness of one's emotion and experience. Health and sickness each have their place, as do joy and sadness. In the end it is the ties of love that remain, and that keep us in each other's hearts.

Health is so much more than the absence of disease.

Glossary

AMINO ACIDS: The molecular building blocks of proteins and peptides.

ANTIBACTERIAL: Any agent that either destroys or stops the replication of bacteria.

ANTIBIOTIC: Literally means "against life"; medicines designed to destroy, or stop the replication of, bacteria. *Not effective against viruses.*

ANTIBODIES: Proteins made by B cells of the immune system in response to the presence in the body of a foreign invader, which specifically seek out and label only this particular invader, thereby enabling its destruction by other immune system components.

ANXIETY: A state of stress generated by remembered or anticipated stress in the absence of an actual stressful situation. In other words, stress.

BACTERIA: Microscopic unicellular organisms found everywhere, that "range from the harmless or beneficial to the intensely virulent and lethal." [*]

DNA: Deoxyribonucleic acid: the molecular substance of genetic material that is passed on to our children. Also contained in every cell of the body, where it directs, or "codes for," the formation of peptides and proteins from amino acids.

ENDOCRINE: Literally means "internal secretion." A system of organs called "glands" that produce hormones. Includes adrenals, ovaries, testes, pancreas, parathyroid, pineal, pituitary, thymus, and thyroid glands.

---

[*] Source: The New International Webster's Comprehensive Dictionary of the English Language Encyclopedia Edition (1996). Naples, FL, USA: Trident Press International.

ENDOTOXIN: A harmful substance released when certain bacteria are destroyed, against which the host is unable to produce an antidote. In this book, also refers to any internally generated product that is not successfully eliminated.

ENERGY: In traditional Chinese medicine energy is also known as "Qi" (pronounced "chee"). Qi, or vital energy, is believed to flow through the body, regulating a person's spiritual, emotional, mental, and physical balance.* Energy is the basic distinguishing characteristic of living things and is generated by living cells.

ENZYME: A short-lived molecule, usually a protein, that accelerates or otherwise enables a biochemical process taking place very near to where the enzyme is produced; usually does not involve transportation by the blood.

EXOTOXIN: A harmful substance made and excreted by an invading organism, in the absence of which its presence would not be harmful. In this book, also refers to any toxic material introduced by inhalation, ingestion, or by direct skin contact.

GALL BLADDER: Waste products cleaned from blood by the liver, along with bile salts (which aid digestion and are produced in the liver) collect in the gall bladder for subsequent delivery into the start of the small intestine, just beyond the stomach.

HEALTH: Health may be viewed as that which enhances the well-being of an individual or population. Defined by the World Health Organisation this way: "Health is a state of complete physical, mental, and social well-being and not merely the absence of disease or infirmity."**

HORMONES: Complex molecules produced in the endocrine glands and secreted into the bloodstream, which carries them to another place in the body where they have an effect. The production of a hormone is often regulated by other hormones, and also by products of its action—which is known as "feedback" control. Hormones can circulate in the bloodstream for some time. Hormones communicate via energy codes and messages read by receptors in cells throughout the body.

---

* Source: MedicineNet.com: www.medterms.com/script/main/alphaidx.asp?p=q_dict.
** World Health Organisation: www.who.org.

GLOSSARY

IMMUNITY: Protection against disease-producing entities by formation of antibodies and other types of substances; a result of exposure to the entities themselves.

LIVER: An organ in the abdomen through which blood from the digestive system passes first. Nutrients are separated from waste products of metabolism here. Nutrients are returned to the blood to be circulated to the rest of the body, while unneeded or harmful substances are delivered back into the small intestine by way of the gall bladder.

LYMPH NODE: A collection of B cells, which produce antibodies; lymph nodes are scattered throughout the body, and are concentrated in places where foreign invaders are likely to be found. The nodes are connected to each other by a system of channels known as "lymphatics."

NEUROTOXIN: A substance that is harmful or lethal to cells of the brain or nerve cells.

NEUROTRANSMITTERS: Substances produced and secreted by brain and nerve cells that bind to receptors of other nearby nervous system cells, signaling a change in the second cell.

ORGANIC: In this book, refers to food grown without the use of synthetic pesticides and fertilizers. ["Organic" is also a term in chemistry referring to carbon-based substances that are (or have once been) alive. "Inorganic" usually refers to materials that have never been alive but that do occur on and in the earth and, indeed, in the universe. Some confusion has been generated by the attempt to characterise "organic" substances as harmless or beneficial and "inorganic" and synthetic (man-made) ones as harmful. Unfortunately, there is no such easy guideline. Many "organic" substances are quite toxic and many "inorganic" or synthetic materials are quite harmless.]

PANCREAS: An organ in the abdomen that produces insulin (an important molecule required for the utilization of food) and also many enzymes used for digestion.

PATHOGEN: Any substance that causes disease.

PATHOLOGY: The study of disease.

PEPTIDE: A very small molecule consisting of two or a few amino acids joined together. Many neurotransmitters are peptides.

PROBIOTIC: Literally means "enhancing life"; in this book refers to beneficial bacteria residing in the digestive tract.

PROTEIN: Chains of amino acids; the molecular substance of enzymes and many other components of life; an essential element of the diet.

RECEPTORS: Molecules on every cell of one's body that respond to chemical messengers like enzymes, antibodies, or even other cells. Binding of one of these by a receptor signals the cell to begin some action (often the internal production of another chemical substance).

STRESS: Any life event ("good" or "bad") that requires change or adaptation.

SYNTHETIC: Made by humans, not found in nature.

SPLEEN: An organ in the abdomen filled with B cells of the immune system, through which blood is circulated.

THYMUS: An endocrine gland in the chest that is part of the immune system. It is in the thymus that lymphocytes mature, multiply, and become T-cells. (That is why they are called T-cells: T for thymus.) It is quite large in the child and becomes proportionately smaller, and less active, in the adult.

References and Author's Notes

CHAPTER 2 — HAPPY, HEALTHY CHILDREN

1. Rhea, W. (1996). Notes on lecture at the Institute of Functional Medicine's "Toxicity '96" Conference, Sea World Nara Resort, Noosa, Queensland, AU.

CHAPTER 3 — INDIVIDUAL DIFFERENCES

1. Retold in: Brennan, J. (1967). *One Solitary Voice*. White Plains, NY, USA: self-published.

CHAPTER 4 — GROWTH AND DEVELOPMENT: MY WORLD

1. Santrock, J.W. (1996). *Child Development*. Madison, WI, USA: Brown and Benchmark.

2. Trout, S. (1996). *To See Differently*. Alexandria, VA, USA: Three Roses Press.

3. Goleman, D. (1995). *Emotional Intelligence*. London, UK: Bloomsbury Publishing.

4. Francis D.D., et al. (2002). Environmental enrichment reverses the effects of maternal separation on stress reactivity. *J. Neuroscience 22(18)*, 7840–7843.

    From notes taken at the Metagenics Seminar, "Management of Childhood Illness," in Launceston, Tasmania, AU, March, 2003.

5. Dawkins, R. (1998). *Unweaving the Rainbow*. London, UK: Allen Lane.

6. Hock, D. (1999). *The Birth of the Chaordic Age*. San Francisco, CA, USA: Berrett-Koehler Publishers, Inc.

7. Parent's Handbook. (1992). *Roots and Wings: Raising Resilient Children.* Hazelden Publishing and Educational Services: Hazelden Press.

   Information available online at: www.hazelden.org/OA_HTML/ ibeCCtpItmDspRte.jsp?a=b&item=1813. Note: *Roots and Wings* is a multiformat, interactive learning program for parents that combines effective parenting skills with an exploration of family standards on alcohol and other drug use.

CHAPTER 5 — STRUCTURE AND FUNCTION

1. Diamond, J. (1979). *Your Body Doesn't Lie.* New York, NY, USA: Warner Books.

2. Pert, C. (1999). *Molecules of Emotion: The Science Behind Mind–Body Medicine.* New York, NY, USA: Touchstone.

3. Hohaus, L. (2004). *Aging and Memory.* Interview of director of the Memory Clinic, Grigriffin University, Queensland, AU, by Julie McCrossin, heard on ABC Radio's national "Life Matters" program June 8.

CHAPTER 6 — TOO MUCH, TOO LITTLE

1. Fromm, E. (1981). *To Have or To Be.* New York, NY, USA: Bantam Books.

2. Alexander, P. (1994). *It Could Be Allergy and It Can Be Cured.* Dee Why, New South Wales, AU: Ethicare Books.

3, 4, 5, 6, 7. Chopra, Deepak. (1991). *Perfect Weight.* New York, NY: Harmony Books.

8. Porter, R. (1997). *Of Greatest Benefit to Mankind: A Medical History of Humanity from Antiquity to the Present.* London, UK: HarperCollins Publishers.

9. Brennan, B. (1988). *Hands of Light: A Guide to Healing Through the Human Energy Field.* New York, NY, USA: Bantam Books.

10. Taylor, F., Krohn, J., Larson E.M. (2000). *Allergy Relief and Prevention: A Practical Encyclopedia.* Point Roberts, WA, USA: Hartley and Marks Publishers.

REFERENCES AND AUTHOR'S NOTES

CHAPTER 7 — ASSESSMENT

1. Walter E. (ed). (2004). *Cambridge Advanced Learner's Dictionary*. Cambridge, UK: Cambridge University Press.

    Barnhart, C.L., Barnhart, R.K. (eds). (1987). *The World Book Dictionary*. Chicago, IL, USA: Doubleday & Company, Inc.

2. Glanze, W.D., Anderson, K.N., Anderson, L.E. (eds). (1990). *Mosby's Medical, Nursing and Allied Health Dictionary, Third Edition*. St. Louis, MO, USA: The C.V. Mosby Company.

3. Omura, Y. (1985). A new, simple, non-invasive imaging technique of internal organs and various cancer tissues using extended principles of the "Bi-Digital O-Ring Test" without using expensive imaging instruments or exposing the patient to any undesirable radiation—Part I. *Acupuncture and Electro-Therapeutics Research 10*, 255–277.

    Scofield, A. (1989). Shamanism, Healing and the Dowsing Tradition. *J. Brit. Soc. Dowsers, 33*(223), 423.

    Note: More information about Dr. Omura and his test is available on the World Wide Web: International College of Acupuncture & Electrotherapeutics (www.icaet.org); International Bi-Digital O-Ring Test Medical Society (http://bdort.net).

4. Note: Pulsating Energy Resonance Therapy (PERT as it is known in scientific circles) is becoming recognised with over 10,000 scientific studies published. It is mainly recognised in Europe but has made its way into the West in recent years.

    Plattner, J., Geber, R.G. (2003). Energy—Source of Life and Health: Health and Healing through Pulsating Energy Resonance Therapy (PERT). Perth Western Australia, AU. *Available online at: www.medec.com.au/index.php?id=18*.

    Note: The point is made that for better or worse we are increasingly affected by these invisible influences. How much wiser to use them for good rather than ignore them and pretend they have no effect on human health!

Heimes, D. (2001). *Resonance/Earth Rays/EMR/ER*. Notes from International Conference of Functional Medicine, presented by Integrated Functional Medicine Pty Ltd, Melbourne, Victoria, AU.

5. Cohen, M. (2001). *Bio-Energetics and Basic Science: Bringing Together Ancient and Modern Concepts.* Notes on lecture at Energy Medicine Conference presented by FIT (Institute of Functional Medicine) at Melbourne, Victoria, AU. April.

Note: I attended a three-day conference on Energy Medicine presented by FIT (Institute of Functional Medicine) at Melbourne, Victoria, AU in April 2001. The Vega equipment was introduced and Prof. Cohen was one of the presenters. The following references were provided.

Chen, K.G. (1996). Applying quantum interference to EDST medicine testing. *IEEE Engineering in Medicine and Biology,* June, 58–63.

Ketalris, C.H., Weiner, J.M., Heddle, R.J., Stuckey, M.S., Yan, K.W. (1991). Vega testing in the diagnosis of allergic conditions. *Med. J. Aust., 155(2),* 113-114.

Mardetko, D. (2001). *Diagnostic and Therapeutic Basics for Modern Holistic Medicine.* Notes on lecture at Energy Medicine Conference, FIT (Institute of Functional Medicine) at Melbourne, Victoria, AU. April.

Szopinski, J., Pantowitz, D., Jaros, G.G. (1998) Diagnostic accuracy of organ electrodermal diagnostics: A pilot study. *S. Afr. Med. J., 88(2),* 146-150.

Tsuei, J., Lam, F.M.K., Chou, P. (1996). Clinical applications of EDST, with an investigation of the organ-meridian relationship. *IEEE Engineering in Medicine and Biology, 16(5),* 415-419.

REFERENCES AND AUTHOR'S NOTES

CHAPTER 8 — SYSTEMS OVERVIEW

1. Pert, C. (1999). *Molecules of Emotion: The Science Behind Mind–Body Medicine.* New York, NY, USA: Touchstone.

2. Tortora, G.J., Grabowski, S.R. (1993). *Principles of Anatomy and Physiology 7th Edition.* New York, NY, USA: Harper Collins Life Sciences.

3. Bengmark, S. (2002). Gut Microbial Ecology in Critical Illness: Is There a Role for Prebiotics, Probiotics and Symbiotics? *Curr. Opinion Crit. Care (2),* 145–151.

    Cited in training manual for Metagenics Seminar, "Management of Childhood Illness," in Launceston, Tasmania, AU, March, 2003.

    Taylor, F., Krohn, J., Larson, E.M. (2000). *Allergy Relief and Prevention: A Practical Encyclopedia.* Point Roberts, WA, USA: Hartley and Marks Publishers.

    Bland, J. (1995). Psychoneuro-Nutritional Medicine: An Advancing Paradigm. *Alternative Therapies in Health & Medicine, 1(2),* 22–27.

    Paper presented at the Third International Symposium on Functional Medicine, Vancouver, BC, Canada, 1996.

4. Note: Amount of water required for a child: Average daily water intake for an adult in a temperate climate is about two litres per day. A child would need proportionally less. One must also take into consideration perspiration, times of fever or illness, and exposure to sun or toxins. Any additional stress on the systems would benefit by an increase of pure water intake. Extrapolating from this basic amount, a small child would need approximately 750 ml to 1 litre and an older child about 1 to 1.5 litres daily.

    Koch, M. (1984). *Laugh With Health.* New York, NY, USA : Holt, Rheinhart & Winston.

    Tortora, G.J., Grabowski, S.R. (1993). *Principles of Anatomy and Physiology, 7th Edition.* New York, NY, USA: Harper Collins Life Sciences.

CHAPTER 9 — NUTRITION

1. Wold, A.E., et al. (2000). Breastfeeding and the intestinal microflora of the infant—Implications for protection against infectious diseases. *Adv. Exp. Med. Biol. 478*, 77–93.

   Santrock, J.W. (1996). *Child Development (7th edition)*. Dubuque, IA, USA: Brown & Benchmark Publishers.

2. Thurgood, A. (2003). "Childhood Illnesses." Notes taken at the Metagenics Seminar, "Management of Childhood Illness," in Launceston, Tasmania, AU. March.

3. Wold, A.E. (1998). The Hygiene Hypothesis Revised: Is the Rising Frequency of Allergy due to Changes in the Intestinal Flora? *Allergy 53, Suppl. 46*, 20–25.

4. Bengmark, S. (2000). Colonic Food: Pre- and Probiotics. *Amer. J. Gastrolenterology 95, Suppl 1*, S 5–7.

5. Bender, A., et al. (2001). Colonic fermentation as affected by antibiotics and acidic pH: Application of an *in vitro* model. *J. Gastroenterology 39(11)*, 911–918.

6. Glanze, W.D., Anderson, K.N., Anderson, L.E. (eds). (1990). *Mosby's Medical, Nursing and Allied Health Dictionary, Third Edition*. St. Louis, MO, USA: The C.V. Mosby Company.

7. Renz, H., et al. (2002). The bi-directional capacity of bacterial antigens to modulate allergy and asthma. *Eur. Respir. J. 19*, 158–171.

   Gehring, U., et al. (2001). Exposure to Endotoxin Decreases the Risk of Atopic Eczema in Infancy: A Cohort Study. *J. Allergy Clin. Immunology 108(5)*, 847–854.

8. "Advise governments to safeguard the effectiveness of vital drugs and ensure their life-saving capacity remains available to future generations."

   Quoted from: *Antimicrobial resistance.* World Health Organisation Fact Sheet No. 194. (Revised Jan. 2002). *Full text available online at www.who.int/entity/medicines_technologies/facts/en/.*

9. Hall, R.H. (1984). *Food for Nought: The Decline in Nutrition.* Hagerstown Maryland, USA: Harper and Row.

10. Gill, H.S., et al. (2000). Enhancement of natural and acquired immunity by Lactobacillus ramnosus (HN001), Lactobacillus acidophilus (HN017) and Bifidobacterium lactis (HN019). *Br. J. Nutr. 83(2),* 167–176.

11. Dengate, S. (1998). *Fed Up.* Milsons Point, NSW, AU: Random House.

12. Davies, S., and Stewart, A. (1987). *Nutritional Medicine: The Drug-free Guide to Better Family Health.* London, UK: Pan Books.

CHAPTER 10 — PROTECTION

1. "Breast milk contains 300 mg of calcium per quart and cow's milk has 1,200 mg per quart, yet infants absorb more calcium from breast milk."

    Taylor, F., Krohn, J., Larson, E.M. (2000). *Allergy Relief and Prevention.* Point Roberts, WA, USA: Hartley & Marks Publishers, page 116.

2. Mazari, L., et al. (1998). Nutritional influences on immune response in healthy aged persons. *Mechanisms of Aging and Development 104(1),* 25–40.

    Notes taken at the Metagenics Seminar, "Clinical Solutions for Immune Disorders," in Launceston, Tasmania, AU, 2002.

    Sprietsma J.E. (1999). Modern diets and diseases: NO-zinc balance. Th1, zinc, nitrogen monoxide collectively protect against viruses, AIDS, auto-immunity, diabetes, allergies, asthma, infectious diseases, atherosclerosis and cancer. *Med. Hypotheses 53(1),* 6–16.

    Notes taken at the Metagenics Seminar, "Clinical Solutions for Immune Disorders," in Launceston, Tasmania, AU, 2002.

3. Renz, H., et al. (2002). The Bi-directional Capacity of Bacterial Antigens to Modulate Allergy and Asthma. *Eur. Respir. J. 19,* 158–171.

    Notes taken at the Metagenics Seminar, "Management of Childhood Illness," in Launceston, Tasmania, AU, March, 2003.

4. Schaechtern, M., Medoff, G., Schlessinger, D. (1989). *Mechanisms of Microbial Disease.* Baltimore, MD, USA: Williams & Wilkins.

5. Bengmark, S. (2002). Gut Microbial Ecology in Critical Illness: Is There a Role for Prebiotics, Probiotics and Synbiotics? *Curr. Opinion Crit. Care (2),* 145–151.

   Notes taken at the Metagenics Seminar, "Management of Childhood Illness," in Launceston, Tasmania, AU, March, 2003.

6. Davies, S., and Stewart, A. (1987). *Nutritional Medicine: The Drug-free Guide to Better Family Health.* London, UK: Pan Books.

7. Gill, H.S., et al. (2001). Dietary probiotic supplementation enhances natural killer cell activity in the elderly. *J. Clin. Immunol 21(4),* 264–271.

   Notes taken at the Metagenics Seminar, "Clinical Solutions for Immune Disorders," in Launceston, Tasmania, AU, 2002.

8. Davies, S., and Stewart, A. (1987). *Nutritional Medicine: The Drug-free Guide to Better Family Health.* London, UK: Pan Books.

9, 10, 11. Renz, H., et al. (2002). The Bi-directional Capacity of Bacterial Antigens to Modulate Allergy and Asthma. *Eur. Respir. J. 19,* 158–171.

   Notes taken at the Metagenics Seminar, "Management of Childhood Illness," in Launceston, Tasmania, AU, March, 2003.

12. Van der Holden, V.H.J., et al. (2001). Selective development of a strong Th2 cytokine profile in high-risk children who develop atopy: Risk factors and regulatory role of IFN-y, IL-4 and IL-10. *Clinical and Experimental Allergy 31,* 997–1006.

   Renz, H., et al. (2002). The Bi-directional Capacity of Bacterial Antigens to Modulate Allergy and Asthma. *Eur. Respir. J. 19,* 158–171.

   Notes taken at the Metagenics Seminar, "Management of Childhood Illness," in Launceston, Tasmania, AU, March, 2003.

13. Warner, J.A., Warner, J.O. (2000). Early life events in allergic sensitisation. *Br. Med. Bull. 56(4),* 883–893.

CHAPTER 11 — COMMUNICATION

1. Pert, C. (1999). *Molecules of Emotion: The Science Behind Mind–Body Medicine.* New York, NY, USA: Touchstone.

2. Goleman, D. (1995). *Emotional Intelligence.* London, UK: Bloomsbury Publishing.

3. Pert, C. (1999). *Molecules of Emotion: The Science Behind Mind–Body Medicine.* New York, NY, USA: Touchstone.

CHAPTER 12 — DETOX

1, 2. Buist, R. (1990). *Food Chemical Sensitivity.* North Ryde New South Wales (NSW), AU: Angus and Robertson.

3. Dengate, S. (1998). *Fed Up.* Milsons Point, NSW, AU: Random House.

4. Rhea, W. (1996). Notes on lecture at the Institute of Functional Medicine's "Toxicity '96" Conference, Sea World Nara Resort, Noosa, Queensland, AU.

CHAPTER 13 — STRESS

1. Glanze, W.D., Anderson, K.N., Anderson, L.E. (eds). (1990). *Mosby's Medical, Nursing and Allied Health Dictionary, Third Edition.* St. Louis, MO, USA: The C.V. Mosby Company.

2. Greenberg, J.S. (2002). *Comprehensive Stress Management.* New York, NY, USA: McGraw Hill Higher Education.

3. Koffman, O. (2002). The role of prenatal stress in the etiology of developmental behavioural disorders—review. *Neurosc. Biobehav. Rev. 26,* 457–470.

Notes taken at the Metagenics Seminar, "Management of Childhood Illness," in Launceston, Tasmania, AU, March, 2003.

4. Goleman, D. (1995). *Emotional Intelligence*. London, UK: Bloomsbury Publishing.

   Francis, D.D., et al. (1999). The Role of Corticotropin-Releasing Factor-Norepinephrine Systems in Mediating the Effects of Early Experience on the Development of Behavioural and Endocrine Response to Stress. *Society of Biological Psychiatry 46*, 1151–1166.

   Notes taken at the Metagenics Seminar, "Management of Childhood Illness," in Launceston, Tasmania, AU, March, 2003.

5. Sapolsky, Robert M. (1994). *Why Zebras Don't Get Ulcers: An Updated Guide to Stress, Stress-Related Diseases, and Coping*. New York, NY. Henry Holt & Company.

6. Koffman, O. (2002). The role of prenatal stress in the etiology of developmental behavioural disorders—review. *Neurosc. Biobehav. Rev. 26*, 457–470.

   Notes taken at the Metagenics Seminar, "Management of Childhood Illness," in Launceston, Tasmania, AU, March, 2003.

7. Merson, J. (2001). *Stress: The Causes, the Costs and the Cures*. Sydney, New South Wales, AU: ABC (Australian Broadcasting Corporation) Books.

CHAPTER 14 — WISER CHOICES

1. Payne, R. (2002). *A Framework for Understanding Poverty*. Highlands, TX, USA: aha! Process, Inc.

About the Author

Ellen Allen has operated a clinic for children since 1983, first in Western Australia and now in Tasmania, Australia.

Ellen received a Bachelor of Science degree from Fordham University, NY, in 1968 and the ND (Diploma of Naturopathy) in 1983 at Dunn's Herbal Clinic in Western Australia. She earned a post-graduate diploma in Clinical Nutrition with R. Buist at the International Academy of Nutrition in Sydney, Australia, in 1996. In 2001 she obtained the Advanced Diploma of Naturopathy, as well as a post-graduate certificate in Traditional Chinese Medicine at Cathay Herbal Labs, which is associated with Zheijing University, China (PRC). In 2003 she was granted a post-graduate diploma in Art Therapy by Dr. Cornelia Elbrecht of Melbourne, Australia. She is a member of the Australian Traditional Medicine Society (ATMS) and the Australian Naturopathic Practitioners Association (ANPA).

After being introduced to basic concepts of energy healing, Ellen developed a system that has evolved over the past 15 years into a quick and effective therapy that deals with energy balance, effects of excessive stress, and physical and behavioural symptoms. The theory operates on the premise that excessive stress blocks healing processes, and that clearing these blocks allows natural repair to occur. She does not treat medical conditions as such, but focuses on supporting function. Ellen conducts her practice within this framework, drawing on skills from her training in several other traditions.

Ellen participated as one of a panel of experts in the ABC (Australian Broadcasting Corporation) television series "Second Opinion," addressing the topic of chronic fatigue syndrome on 19 April 2005 and attention deficit disorder on 7th June 2005. "Second Opinion" provides an excellent forum for alternative and medical practitioners to discuss their views on different conditions; enhanced understanding between health providers of all persuasions can only serve to benefit those suffering from illness.

ORDER FORM

Please send me ___ copy/copies of *Growing Healthy Children* at $14.95 per book. Enclosed is payment for:

    Books $ _____

    Shipping $ _____ ($4.50 first book + $2.00 each additional book)

    Subtotal $ _____

    Sales tax $ _____ (6.25% Texas residents only)

    Total $ _____

Ship-to Address (no post office boxes, please)

Name _____

Organization _____

Address _____

_____

Phone _____

E-mail _____

Method of Payment

PO # _____

Credit card type _____ Exp. _____

Credit card # _____

Check # _____

    Order online at: www.amazon.com
    or
    Send this form to: RubyFire
                                 P.O. Box 727
                                 Highlands, TX 77562-0727
                                 fax 281-426-8705

Thank you for your order!